Institutionalizing Assisted Reproductive Technologies

Reproductive medicine has been very successful at developing new therapies in recent years and people having difficulties conceiving have more options available to them than ever before. These developments have led to a new institutional landscape emerging and this innovative volume explores how health and social structures are being developed and reconfigured to take into account the increased use of assisted reproductive technologies, such as IVF treatments.

Using Sweden as a central case study, it explores how the process of institutionalizing new assisted reproductive technologies includes regulatory agencies, ethical committees, political bodies and discourses, scientific communities, patient and activists groups, and entrepreneurial activities in the existing clinics and new entrants to the industry. It draws on new theoretical developments in institutional theory and outlines how health innovations are always embedded in social relations including ethical, political, and financial concerns.

This book will be of interest to advanced students and academics in health management, science and technology studies, the sociology of health and illness and organizational theory.

Alexander Styhre is Professor and Chair of Organization Theory and Management at the University of Gothenburg, Sweden.

Rebecka Arman is Assistant Professor of Organization Theory and Management at the University of Gothenburg, Sweden.

Routledge Studies in the Sociology of Health and Illness

Available titles include:

Dimensions of Pain
Humanities and Social Science Perspectives
Edited by Lisa Folkmarson Käll

Aging Men, Masculinities and Modern Medicine
Edited by Antje Kampf, Barbara L. Marshall and Alan Petersen

Disclosure in Health and Illness
Mark Davis and Lenore Manderson

Caring and Well-being
A Lifeworld Approach
Kathleen Galvin and Les Todres

Systems Theory and the Sociology of Health and Illness
Observing Healthcare
Edited by Morten Knudsen and Werner Vogd

Complaints, Controversies and Grievances in Medicine
Edited by Jonathan Reinarz and Rebecca Wynter

The Public Shaping of Medical Research
Patient Associations, Health Movements and Biomedicine
Edited by Peter Wehling and Willy Viehöver

Giving Blood
The Institutional Making of Altruism
Edited by Johanne Charbonneau and André Smith

Health, Food and Social Inequality
Critical Perspectives on the Supply and Marketing of Food
Carolyn Mahoney

Institutionalizing Assisted Reproductive Technologies

The role of science, professionalism and regulatory control

Alexander Styhre and Rebecka Arman

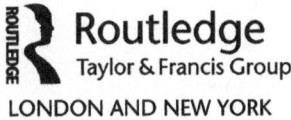

Routledge
Taylor & Francis Group

LONDON AND NEW YORK

First published 2016
by Routledge
4 Park Square, Milton Park, Abingdon, Oxon OX14 4RN
605 Third Avenue, New York, NY 10017

First issued in paperback 2023

Routledge is an imprint of the Taylor & Francis Group, an informa business

British Library Cataloguing-in-Publication Data
A catalogue record for this book is available from the British Library

Library of Congress Cataloging in Publication Data
Names: Styhre, Alexander, author. | Arman, Rebecka, 1976- , author.Title: Institutionalizing assisted reproductive technologies : the role of science, professionalism, and regulatory control / Alexander Styhre and Rebecka Arman.Other titles: Routledge studies in the sociology of health and illness.Description: Abingdon, Oxon ; New York, NY : Routledge, 2016. | Series: Routledge studies in the sociology of health and illness | Includes bibliographical references and index.Identifiers: LCCN 2015037530| ISBN 9781138806214 (hbk) | ISBN 9781315751795 (ebk)Subjects: | MESH: Reproductive Techniques, Assisted.Classification: LCC RG133.5 | NLM WQ 208 | DDC 616.6/92--dc23LC record available at http://lccn.loc.gov/2015037530

ISBN: 978-1-138-80621-4 (hbk)
ISBN: 978-1-315-75179-5 (ebk)
ISBN: 978-0-367-22398-4 (pbk)

DOI: 10.4324/9781315751795

Typeset in Times New Roman
by Saxon Graphics Ltd, Derby

Publisher's Note
The publisher has gone to great lengths to ensure the quality of this reprint but points out that some imperfections in the original copies may be apparent.

Contents

PART III
Institutionalizing ART **165**

Preface

In 2013, we published the research monograph *Reproductive Medicine and the Life Sciences in the Contemporary Economy*, which was the outcome from our joint work to explore how one of the most widespread and appreciated clinical practices based on life science research in universities and research institutes had been established also as a commercial activity. When exploring the social science and organization theory literature addressing assisted reproductive technologies (ART), in vitro fertilization (IVF), and reproductive medicine more broadly, there was a rather limited amount of studies being published. Especially organization theorists and management scholars appeared to be only modestly interested in the commercialization of reproductive medicine taking place over the last few decades since the late 1970s.

In the literature on life science innovation, which initially triggered our interest in this field, there is a constant call for success stories that can justify further investment in both basic research and attract new investors to the field. Unfortunately, as life science innovation is immensely complex and demands very costly clinical trials to safeguard the stock of empirical data demanded to have a new compound or new medical device or technology accepted by regulatory bodies, it is far more likely that life science start-up firms will fail rather than bring the innovation all the way to the market. Given this shortage of exemplary cases of how either individual innovations, or, in our case, an entire scientific field become successful in advancing a new clinical practice, we were surprised to notice the quite meager interest in e.g., reproductive medicine, especially among business school researchers. Instead, we learned, it was feminist scholars who primarily wrote and debated the nature of and benefits and perils of the new reproductive possibilities. While this literature was inspiring to read and certainly added to our work, it contained only a small number of empirical studies of e.g., ART and IVF clinics. We tried our best to identify e.g., ethnographic studies or fieldwork-based studies of IVF clinics, but we could only find a handful of publications.

As we still believe that ART and reproductive medicine are both highly significant as a professional field of expertise, strongly influencing everyday life for millions of sub-fertile women and couples, and because the industry today has a substantial turnover and an impressive growth rate, we decided to continue our research work. While our first volume focused primarily on the work conducted within the clinics – the work conducted by counselors and gynecologists directly encountering the patients, but also the work done by e.g., embryologists working in the laboratories that the regular patients in most cases never visit or get access to – this volume is taking a wider view and includes an analysis of what occurs outside of the clinic. Such sites include regulatory agencies, bioethical committees, activist communities, and university-based reproductive medicine departments, all participating in their own idiosyncratic ways to the advancement of what can be called "reproductive futures."

The overarching theoretical perspective taken in this volume – the first volume emphasized the materiality of the clinical practices, including both gametes and reproductive materials but also the instruments, technologies and devices involved in the creation and transferring of human embryos – is institutional theory. More specifically, we have used the recent literature on *institutional work* and *institutional logics*, which to a higher extent than the "classical" and so-called neo-institutional theory literature emphasize agency, change and innovativeness in organizations and organizational fields. In the parlance of e.g., the institutional work literature, actors involved in further differentiation and refining of practices and/or the regulatory frameworks determining such practices participate in institutional work: they actively inform and shape the institutions (e.g., laws, regulations, medical "golden standards," accounting practices and guidelines, etc.), which if they don't determine, at least effectively set the standards for the legitimate and qualified clinical practices.

Institutional theory is by and large a staple theory in organization and management studies, being one of the most widespread but also most prestigious theoretical perspectives in business school research, but it has frequently been criticized for ignoring or marginalizing the question of agency. In the light of such debates, the literature on institutional work and institutional logics affords some new possibilities for institutional analyses that better explore how change and novelty are initiated and come about. If nothing else, we believe that we have been able to handle our empirical material in meaningful ways on the basis of this literature, and thus being able to add, we hope, to the scholarship on the commercialization and regulation of ART, assisted reproduction, and reproductive medicine as domains for venturing and enterprising.

In addition to the institutional theory, we have also made use of a variety of social science and organization theory sub-genres including science and technology studies, economic sociology, studies informed by feminist theory, neoclassical economic theory references, and a fair share of classic organization theory in this volume. While the volume includes a significant amount of theoretical sections, we have used these references to address our empirical material in ways so that we can bring forward some of the complexities and trade-offs inherent to all professional fields, not the least in the intersection between commerce, life science research, and health care. In this intersection, a variety of institutional logics and competing ideas, norms, and beliefs meet and become entangled, leading to at times, close to irresolvable concerns and debates (e.g., in the case of the legal status and recommendations regarding commercial surrogacy), while in other cases they can be reconciled and brought into at least a temporal harmony (like in the case of Sweden, where public sector health care provisions are quite effectively combined with private clinics). If there is some moral or key learning from this volume (and the study of ART and assisted reproduction at large), it is that the combination of human curiosity (an essential feature of all scientific pursuits), an entrepreneurial culture and attitude (propelling the commercialization process of sound clinical practices), and the most human desire to become parents, together constitutes a strong brew that has greatly expanded the human capacity to intervene in the elementary processes of the biological lives of humans. Therefore, we would welcome more researchers to further extend the scholarship in this domain.

Acknowledgements

The authors would like to thank Terry Clague, Senior Commissioning Editor, Taylor and Francis, Routledge and Grace McInnes, Senior Editor, Health and Social Care, for commissioning this book. Second, we would like to thank the Swedish Research Council (Vetenskapsrådet) for the research grant that financed the research reported in this volume. Third and finally, we are indebted to all the participating researchers, clinicians, company representatives, politicians, agency representatives, and individuals being part of our empirical work. Thank you so much for sharing some of your precious time and your experiences and thoughts with us!

1 Introduction

The science of life and the market for babies

Introduction

The purpose of this research monograph is to examine how a field of expertise is related to and accommodates new innovations, practices, technologies, and concepts that in turn serve to renew and maintain the interest among professional groups, policy-makers and other relevant social groups. This purpose can be divided into two specific objectives:

- To understand the historical development of the clinical therapies and the various practical and ethical issues these therapies give rise to and how they were handled by relevant actors.
- To examine how clinicians, managers, entrepreneurs, and decision-makers actively inform and structure the field of assisted reproduction.

In the contemporary period, human lives are in many ways informed and shaped by the biomedical technosciences producing a variety of therapies, skills, products, services, and procedures wherein the human biological organism is being modified, restored, improved, and enhanced. Social scientists are frequently referencing the seminal work of Michel Foucault on what he refers to as *biopolitics* and *biopower* to underline the generic Foucaultian idea that power/knowledge constitutes an irreducible apparatus (see e.g., Lemke, 2011). In this view and in the case of biomedical technoscience, the growth of therapeutic expertise and skills in medicine and physiology also leads to new possibilities for monitoring and controlling a population, i.e., to make use of new sources of knowledge as a form of *puissance*, "repressive" or "regressive" power. At the same time, Foucault stays true to his Nietzschean convictions and suggests that these apparatuses of biomedical knowledge/power are also productive and enabling, representing a form of *pouvoir*, an "enabling" or "progressive" power that helps humans live better and happier lives.

In addition to the Foucaultian concepts of biopolitics and biopower, there are social scientists that have combined the advancement in biomedical technosciences with increased marketization and financialization and thus view these new power/ knowledge apparatuses as a source of income and the principal driver for various venturing activities. Rose (2007) speaks of the *bioeconomy*, a term that imbricates the science of life and the living with economic and financial pursuits and interests. This sociological term is well aligned with general expectations that the life sciences will take over the role of the manufacturing industry as what would drive economic growth and create job opportunities in the future. In the bioeconomy, economic value, social well-being, and work opportunities are all provided on the basis of expertise in the life sciences and the ability of academic researchers, innovation system agency officers, and venture capital investors to jointly create (small and) expanding companies around research findings in the life sciences.

This volume examines one particular area within the biomedical technosciences: the field of reproductive medicine and its clinical branch assisted reproduction or what is called assisted reproductive technologies (ART). Human infertility and sub-fertility is a growing concern in many parts of the world, both caused by social factors such as the postponement of parenting in many affluent societies, in many cases until the latter 30s, and environmental factors including the concern for low sperm concentration and sperm motility in the case of male infertility, in many cases treated as an effect of environmental factors. It is estimated that around 10 percent of all couples and single women experience infertility problems. Despite this magnitude of the problem and the widespread understanding that involuntary childlessness causes suffering, assisted reproduction practices encounter the common sense objection that "there are already too many babies with no parents or parents that are unable or unwilling to care for them," a declaration which tends to portray assisted reproduction as a form of "luxury medicine," or a concern for primarily financially endowed middle-class individuals in the Western world. Such criticism needs to be unpacked and responded to, but it is noteworthy that this firm belief in reproductive medicine as being a form of luxury health care has managed to penetrate also decision-making communities and qualified actors, leading to researchers operating in this field of expertise experiencing difficulties in attracting research funding. In fact, in many cases, research projects in reproductive medicine need to be associated with other therapeutic areas (e.g., oncology and, in particular, stem cell research and regenerative medicine) to justify ongoing research work.

In addition to this more general common sense objection, reproductive medicine has also been branded by religious, primarily Christian groups, as a field of biomedical technoscience which risks violating the dignity of human life as elementary reproductive materials are being manipulated in clinics and in laboratories. Seemingly paradoxical for some, the "pro-life lobby" dominated by Catholic groups and the American Christian right are not receiving these new reproductive possibilities as favorably as one may think. These technical procedures in their view expand beyond "natural" ways of conceiving a child, i.e., through "unprotected coitus." The "pro-life" agenda thus primarily denote a concern for "naturally conceived life" rather than *all* forms of human life. It is easy to understand that the entire procedure to retrieve eggs, fertilize them in a laboratory setting, and to store them in freezers is something entirely different than the standard reproduction through intercourse, but this criticism can be articulated against virtually any kind of clinical medical practice. There is nothing "natural" about bypass surgery, consuming hypertension drugs, or even using anesthesia during operations, and yet many human beings are deeply thankful for being able to take advantage of these biomedical skills and know-how. In this view, the pro-life objection to reproductive medicine is selective in terms of portraying *some* but not *all* medical practices as unnatural and therefore deplorable or even culpable.

In this volume, reproductive medicine and ART are treated as a field of biomedical technoscience and a health care practice that is embedded in a specific, local but also international institutional setting including legal, regulatory, normative, ethical, political, and financial and economic conditions. These conditions in various ways shape and inform both the research work and the clinical practices. Some of these laws and regulations are based on international agreements including the routines and standards for selecting embryos, while others are locally enacted. As a consequence, there are significant variations across nations and regions, and while, for instance, single women are eligible for IVF in Denmark, they are not in Sweden. In Sweden, moreover, the costs of IVF treatment is roughly one fourth of that of the U.S., the latter being a country that does not provide any public sector and tax-financed IVF therapy as part of the welfare state offering. In many places in the world, including the "infertility belt" in sub-Saharan Africa, few infertile couples are able to pay for the IVF therapy that might help them become parents.

The empirical material reported in Part II of this volume was collected in Sweden, a country renowned for its political commitment to the welfare state, and consequently offering all infertile couples IVF therapies for the first born child. Within the "third way," "mixed economy," or embedded liberalism economic framework of the Scandinavian welfare states, the second child born on the basis of IVF therapy has to be financed individually by the would-be parents. Fortunately, the private IVF clinics in Sweden have very consciously worked to keep the prices at a low level, and today private clinics' IVF therapies are reasonably priced in the range of 33,000 Swedish crowns (around €3,600).

As infertility does not affect everyone, it is still widespread enough to be perceived as a joint social concern as many people know someone or has a family member that have taken advantage of assisted reproduction practices. In addition, ART is a phenomenon that cuts through many social science categories including nature/culture, normal/pathological, natural/artificial, etc., and that aligns various scholarly and professional domains of expertise, including specific fields of medicine (reproductive medicine, gynecology, obstetrics, organ transplant surgery, etc.) and veterinary medicine, law studies, organization and management theory, political science, and what today is referred to as *bioethics*, the study of ethical and moral issues pertaining to the uses of medical science and practices (see e.g., Hedgecoe, 2010). Needless to say, this volume will not be able to cover all areas of relevance for the history and everyday practice of reproductive medicine and ART, but it still seeks to provide a relatively coherent analytical framework including both organization theory and institutional theory in particular

(Chapter 2) and social science studies of reproductive medicine and ART (Chapter 3) to be able to report and frame the empirical material.

The volume also sets out to advance the thesis that reproductive medicine and ART are best understood as what are recursively both shaped and informed by and is shaping and informing the institutional framework wherein it is embedded. In the contemporary era, where everything "bio" is highly praised and treated as both a source of economic and entrepreneurial growth in the stagnating economies of the West and what will create happier, healthier, and longer human lives, reproductive medicine and ART constitute one specific field of expertise and know-how – a knowledge/power assemblage – that has effectively proved its clinical and practical value. Unlike many other biomedical technoscientific concepts including nanotechnology or genomics, reproductive medicine and ART have not only contributed to the growth of the stock of biomedical know-how but have offered a quite straightforward solution to the infertility problems, and today between 3 and 5 percent of all children born in the West are fertilized in the laboratory.

However, the widespread use of ART is a human accomplishment that cannot solely be understood on the basis of the heroic accomplishments of the pioneers and champions of the field but also as a more ongoing collective engagement that includes a variety of actors representing many different interests and organizations. In addition to the sheer organizational complexities of ART practices the literature of relevance for this scholarly pursuit to study and understand the development of reproductive medicine and ART, easily expands in all directions. We have still tried our best to point at the scope of "the problem" of reproductive medicine and ART inasmuch as we try to cover some of the different literatures of relevance for the study. In short, this volume represents a transdisciplinary view of what reproductive medicine and ART are or could be, and how these domains of expertise serve society through being aligned with wider social concerns and interests.

The concept of life and the gospel of the natural

The first major philosophical treatise on biology and the organism is Aristotle's *De Anima*, poorly translated into *On the Soul*, a title that arguably inscribed too much Christian theology into the original Greek term. Nevertheless, in *De Anima*, Aristotle develops an "ontology of life," wherein there is an analytical distinction between *life* and "*something-other-than-life*" – "that-through-which-the-living-is-living" (Thacker, 2010: x. Emphasis in the original). Aristotle introduces the term *psukhē* but distinguishes between, as Thacker (2010: 17) says, *psukhē*-as-principle (the vital component of all life) and *psukhē*-as-manifestation (the living organism). This separation between principle and manifestation has been a standard binary distinction that haunts the life sciences as it creates an ontological distinction between life and non-life. For instance, a virus is treated as a molecule, i.e., the virus is not "life," while a bacteria is treated as a form of organic life. In this Aristotelian view, the living and the force or vitality of life remains separated, yet entangled.

To this day, in the era of information where biological matter is treated as what is basically understood as sequences of informational patterns (e.g., the human genome), the force of life is yet to be explained. Immanuel Kant provided the first "modern" definition of the organism in his *Critique of judgment* (sec. 65, #372) where an organism is defined as a "*self-organizing* being": "*An organized product of nature is one in which every part is reciprocally purpose, [end] and means*. In it nothing is in vain, without purpose" (Kant, [1790] 2005: §66, p. 166. Emphasis in the original). In addition, anticipating the work of e.g., Erwin Schrödinger's *What is life?* (1944), Kant speaks of the "purposive dispositions" or *Anlagen* of the organism, the inherent properties that regulate its self-organizing existence (Bennett, 2010: 71). These two classic philosophical works, of immense importance for the history of ideas, both render life as what is open-ended and what has no end-points; the impulse of life is "[n]ot to reach a terminus but to keep on going" (Ingold, 2010: 98). Therefore, life is change, procreation, and adaptation in the ceaseless process of "coming-to-be" and "passing-away" and – in Aristotle's terms – being in the perpetual state of "development or decomposition" (Thacker, 2010: 251).

Despite this ontology of life recognizing the impulse to change and become, the concept of nature, a derivate term from life and the living, has been institutionalized in human vocabularies as being substantially less fluid and adaptable. In fact, ideas about nature and what is "natural" are part of a lay vocabulary, rooted in common sense thinking, and not always immune to moralist sentiments. "The very word 'natural' is deeply ideological," Hacking (2002: 7) proposes; "From at latest the time of Aristotle, the idea of nature has served as a way to disguise ideology, to appear to be perfectly neutral" (ibid.). The idea of nature as a pristine, separated, and untarnished domain existing outside of human influence is widely popular in lay communities, but such an idealized view of nature poorly represents the "nature" that humans encounter in everyday life situations and that e.g., the biomedical technosciences investigate.

This idealized view of nature clearly separates humans and human pursuits from nature, the environment wherein humans exist, but as Canguilhem (2008) points out, this distinction rests upon the fallacy that such a separation can be accomplished. Instead, Canguilhem (ibid.: 8) writes, "In a sense, nothing is more human than a machine, if it is true that man distinguishes himself from animals through the construction of tools and machines." Humans rarely encounter nature "in the raw," but instead they re-create and modify elements of nature that can be controlled and regulated, ranging from rural landscapes and their fields and plantations, to gardens, and life science laboratory cell lines, etc. In line with this view, Fourcade (2011: 1770) argues, "[n]ature is never nature but an assemblage of relations involving humans and nonhumans." There are few domains where the artifice of recreated nature is more salient than in the life science laboratory, where what Rheinberger (1997) refers to as *experimental systems* serve to mimic controllable elements of nature in order to produce solid scientific data. Fujimura (1996: 31) states:

Scientists 'create' nature in laboratories just as they create 'intelligence' in computers. They create 'nature' along the lines of particular commitments and with particular constraints, just as computer scientists create computer technologies along the lines of particular commitments and with particular constraints. Thus, the boundary between science and technology is blurred.

More importantly, further undermining the moralist belief in nature "in the raw," these experimental systems frequently include the use of "inbred animals, tissue culture materials and methods, and tumor viruses" (Fujimura, 1996: 66) that all serve as "standardized experimental systems" which enable a controlled and regulated environment. For instance, laboratory animals such as the fruitfly (Kohler, 1994) or genetically modified mice (Rader, 2004) are biological organisms that either are capable of reproducing in short cycles or can easily be genetically modified to express e.g., certain genetic qualities. That is, while e.g., genetically modified mice – scientists at times speak of "knock-out mice" in the case where one or a few gene sequences has been eliminated or rendered passive – are quite far from the common sense idea of nature. Instead, they are biological machines engineered to serve their vital role in biomedical experimental systems (Davies, 2013; Lewis et al., 2013; Birke, 2012; For the case of reproductive medicine, see Friese and Clarke, 2013). Simondon (1980: xiv) reminds us that the Greek etymology of the concept of machine renders it "a trick against nature."

If the term machine and all its connotations with inert matter and engineering and materials science poorly capture the qualities of these laboratory animals, the term *monster* may more adequately capture their role. A *teratology*, a "science of monsters" is derived from the Greek *teras*, meaning both "horror" and "marvel," and the term monster comes from the Latin *monstrere*, "to show" (Campbell and Saren, 2010: 159). While the folklore and popular culture is filled with monsters that are scary and with terrifying looks, the monsters of the laboratory have few visible traits on the phenotype level and they look like regular, small, quite cute white mice. Their ability to serve as marvels (for some) or induce horror (for others) lies precisely in their genotype, their manipulated and engineered hereditary material that makes them experimental platforms where research results can be displayed.

Today, there are 2,000–3,000 types of genetically modified mice in the world (Braidotti, 2006: 101). The first and most well-known, the fabled Harvard Onco-Mouse, was the first patented living organism (Murray, 2010; Kevles, 2002), and is one fine example of how these little genetically modified creatures violate the idea of primordial nature. First patented in 1988, Harvard was for several years refused any patents in Europe because European patent law prohibited the patenting of "plant and animal varieties or the essentially biological processes for the production of plants and animals" (Bud, 1993: 216). On the one hand, the representatives of the American University treated the onco-mouse as a biotechnological invention, a form, albeit unusual, of engineered matter, while the European legislators did not recognize these claims. The monstrosity of the onco-mouse thus derives from its ability to transcend and effectively destroy the boundaries between nature and non-nature, naturally occurring species and artifice, natural birth and engineered life.

The laboratory work in the biomedical technosciences thus widely expands outside of what common sense thinking renders as being "natural," and consequently fields of professional expertise such as reproductive medicine and assisted reproduction encounters a skeptical attitude or outright criticism. This hardnosed emphasis on pristine nature and what is "natural" runs counter to much contemporary technoscience and advanced medical practice, but it affects professional fields differently, arguably with reproductive medicine and assisted reproduction being exposed to a higher level as pregnancies, birth, babies, family life, etc. all belong to an intimate sphere demanding privacy. Being able to respond to demands for "natural" processes or "nature-like" conditions must therefore be part of the professional skills in reproductive medicine and assisted reproduction. Common sense thinking and lay beliefs are also part of the most advanced biomedical technosciences.

Where nature is modified and the bioeconomy is created: the concept of markets

One of the key concerns for policy-makers is how the new therapies and products of contemporary biomedical technosciences are to be priced and allocated to increase the utility of initial investments. In many welfare states, there are public sector health care systems providing health care services, while in other countries, most noteworthy the U.S., there is a preference for market solutions to the pricing and matching of supply and demand problems. In either case, the market for health care services is the principal analytical model for the pricing of health care services.

In this setting, it is important to distinguish between the institutionally embedded view of the market of economic sociology and the axiomatic view of markets as a superior processor of information in neoclassical economic theory. Aspers (2010: 1), an economic sociologist, defines a market as "a social structure for the exchange of rights in which offers are evaluated and priced, and compete with one another." While this definition does not say very much about the institutions that embed and legitimize markets, economic sociologists tend to enact the market as an institution per se, and therefore this specific institutionalized form of economic exchanges cannot be taken for granted but must itself be explained: "Institutions are not residual, but are the basic foundations of society. Any sociological explanation of macrolevel phenomena should include institutional factors," Roy (1997: 170) argues. As a consequence, as opposed to the neoclassical economic theory view of the market, the markets-as-institutions view also distinguishes between *processes of valuation* and *processes of pricing*.

For neoclassical economic theory, markets do little more than to price commodities and services, by definition exactly at the point where supply and demand intersect, and consequently the concept of *valuation* is an unnecessary complication that can be spared. For economic sociologists, pricing is the end-point of the process to build an institutional setting wherein commodities and services can be traded, and the various legal, moral, normative rules and regulations that constitute markets need to be put into place. "'Economy' refers not just to the quantitative measures of productivity or profit, but also to the *regimes of value*, both material and symbolic, that form the theatre of political articulation," Sunder Rajan (2012: 19) emphasizes. For instance, in order to create a legal framework for the trade of a particular commodity, there needs to be a valuation of the commodity prior to the actual pricing of the commodity. To use the case of Fourcade (2011), examining how the courts in France and the U.S. value nature in the face of the unfortunate event of oil spills damaging coastal areas, "nature" cannot simply be treated as any commodity that can be priced on a market, but instead a variety of legal and institutional factors including ownership rights, the costs for cleaning the oil spill, the environmental effects on wildlife and water quality, and so forth, need to be determined. First, when these "rules of the game" are established, making it possible for various actors to determine costs, risks, and benefits, there can be a market for, say, transportation services in the fuel industry. Expressed differently, when the commodity is priced on an open market through bids on a particular item, a series of processes of valuation has already taken place.

In addition, neoclassical economic theory assumes that markets are the most efficient mechanism for pricing commodities, and economists tend to believe that the creation of open markets per se – where free competitions reward cost-reducing or differentiating innovations in both the commodity per se and the production process – increases the efficiency of economic transactions and the economy at large. Economic sociologists, in contrast, treating markets as being embedded in institutions, think of economic growth and economic stability as the outcome from stable political, legal, regulatory, and civil institutions that enables long-term predictability (Fligstein and Choo, 2005: 67). In addition, high-growth economies are characterized by a state administration that does not seek too much rent, i.e., "[n]ot so corrupt that payoff, bribes, and extortion are regular ways of doing business," that helps resolve or mediate class struggle and capital–labor relations, and that lets "private actors accumulate wealth, and generally provide for public order" (ibid.: 67–68). While neoclassical economic theory thinks of the market as accomplishing these goals, economic sociologists believe it is the comprehensive institutional environment, effectively balancing various interest and short- and long-term goals, that provides the possibilities for economic prosperity.

These general differences between neoclassical and sociological views of the market become visible when the market is proposed as a general solution to the allocation of resources, which in turn is embedded in moral or ethical concerns, including, as in our case, the market for babies, embryos, and gametes (reproductive cells). While the market may price virtually any commodity through its supply and demand mechanism, it is not evident that human beings want to encourage anything to become marketable commodities. Marriage, for instance, has historically been treated as an economic exchange between families operating under the norms of exogamy and the incest taboo – the latter one of the few universals of human culture (Lévi-Strauss, 1985: 34–35) – both in the rural setting and in the bourgeoisie of the cities and towns. But marriage was more of an "arrangement between families" than an open market operation, and today, when there are more opportunities for an individualized lifestyle and where women are full legal subjects no longer subsumed under patriarchal traditions and authority, romantic love is the predominant ideology and explanatory factor for how marriages are organized (Luhmann, 1986; Simmel, 1984).

A similar case would be the market for children and assisted reproduction services, discussed below, being part of a sphere of intimacy that poorly lends itself to open-market transactions (Zelizer, 2005). At the same time, some commentators claim that a market for babies and assisted reproduction services would be able to solve a series of problems and issues, leading to both better supply of gametes (and human eggs in particular) and fewer abortions in the case of more efficient markets for adopted children.

The baby market and the baby business

One of the most controversial consequences of assisted reproduction technologies and the clinical practices derived from reproductive medicine is that these practices can isolate the different biological processes and entities from one another – adhering to what Suchman (2007: 3) speaks of as an "ontology of separateness" wherein separate things "need to be joined together" – and thereafter render them subject to market transactions. What has been called the *baby market* (Goodwin, 2010) or a *baby business* (Spar, 2006) is therefore created on the basis of technoscientific biomedical competencies. For many commentators, the creation of such markets is problematic as money exchanges tend to represent what economic sociologist Viviana Zelizer (2011: 34) speaks of as a "profanation" of what belong to the sacred genera. The hostility towards the idea of a market for babies of the reproductive materials and services that precede them is rooted in the Aristotelian idea that money is "sterile" (De Roover, 1974c: 344). In addition, money as a public exchange medium, for many per se a source of greed and opportunistic behavior, poorly blends with the intimacy of human reproduction, historically being part of private family life: "[M]oney and intimacy represent contradictory principles whose intersection generates conflict, confusion, and corruption. Thus people debate passionately the propriety of compensated egg donations, sale of blood and human organs, purchased child care or elder care, and wages for housewives" (Zelizer, 2005: 27). At the same time as there is a taboo against receiving money for a baby, as such transactions would violate the "prohibition against the relinquishment of parental rights in exchange of compensation" (Krawiec, 2010: 41), there are millions of dollars changing hands annually in baby markets – in adoption agencies, in sperm banks, in egg agencies, and in IVF clinics. Apparently, there is a quite pragmatic attitude towards baby markets and therefore the concept of market would deserve some systematic analysis.

The idea of a "market for babies" was first introduced in an article published by Elizabeth Landes and Richard Posner in 1978. Richard Posner is today a judge on the United States Court of Appeals for the Seventh Circuit in Chicago, nominated by President Ronald Reagan in 1981. Posner is widely associated with a libertarian tradition of thinking, and at times treated as an ultra-orthodox defender of free-market capitalism by his critics. In their seminal paper, Landes and Posner (1978) speak of the adoption of children and abortion rates, but do not mention assisted reproduction technologies at all, still not an effective therapy by the time of the publication of the article. Landes and Posner (ibid.: 325) claim that the increased availability of contraceptives and abortion has not reduced the number of "illegitimate births" and points at the "thousands of children in foster care" as being indicative of a poorly functioning "market for babies." Landes and Posner (ibid.) therefore propose a de-regulation of this "market," eliminating the "monopolization" of a few adoption agencies:

> We believe that the large number of children in foster care is, in part, a manifestation of a regulatory pattern that (1) combined restrictions on the sale of babies with the effective monopolization of the adoption market by adoption agencies, and (2) fails to provide effectively for the termination of the natural parents' rights.
>
> (Landes and Posner, 1978: 327)

Using a neoclassical economic theory vocabulary and a calculative rational choice theory line of reasoning, Landes and Posner (1978) speak of "prices," "quality," and "supply" to advance their free-market solution to the "matching problem" leading to both, Landes and Posner (ibid.) argue, higher abortion rates and more children in foster care than necessary. For instance, the children in foster care are, Landes and Posner (ibid.: 327) propose, "comparable to an unsold inventory stored in a warehouse," but if only the "market for babies" would be de-regulated, the "efficiency" would increase, they claim: "There is no reason to believe that prices would be so high where the sale of babies is legalized. On the contrary, prices for children of *equivalent quality* would be much lower" (Landes and Posner, ibid.: 339. Emphasis in the original). In addition, in a "free adoption market," Landes and Posner (ibid.: 343) predict, "some of the 900,000 fetuses aborted in 1974 would have been born and placed for adoption."

While Landes and Posner's (1978) argument is based on an efficiency criteria and the assumption that children and the would-be children of the aborted fetuses can be examined like any other "commodity" amenable to free-market transactions, other commentators have expressed a less rationalist and efficiency-oriented view of the market for babies. Ertman (2010) argues persuasively that a market for gametes (egg and sperm) is justified, that the market for adoption is de facto already in place, and that a market for embryos, similar to that of regulated pharmaceutical drugs should be considered. Ertman (ibid.) advocates what she refers to as (after John Stuart Mill) a "Millian liberalism" as a means to overcome the majority's normative and moral beliefs as a key factor determining the possibilities of individuals to create families of their own:

[M]arket mechanisms provide unique opportunities for law and culture to recognize that people form families in different ways. If state or federal law, rather than the law of supply and demand, determines who can have children using reproductive technologies, then many single and gay people likely will be excluded from this important life experience.

(Ertman, 2010: 23)

In Ertman's (2010) view, the market offers a liberating possibility in terms of enabling minorities (racial, ethnic, and sexual) to escape predominant moral beliefs about what is "natural" and/or socially desirable and what is not. These minorities, by virtue of their numbers, Ertman (ibid.: 23) says, "are unlikely to obtain legal rights and protections through the legislative process – to skirt the majoritarian morality that would otherwise prevent them from forming families." For instance, Ertman says, in the case where one woman decides to donate her eggs to another woman, she would act "altruistically" if the two women are friends, but if they are lovers, certain groups may cease to regard the egg donation as an act of generosity and consider their relationship differently.

For Ertman, in a liberal tradition of thought, the collective has no such right to examine personal relationships and intimacies to determine the legitimacy of such decisions:

Supporters of measures protecting so-called traditional families (and harming so-called nontraditional families) often make moral argument that heterosexuality and two-parent families are natural, relegating others to the category 'unnatural.' *Moral* or *natural* are flexible terms that carry multiple meanings such as 'inevitable' ('it's only natural') or 'mandated by either biology or God' (i.e., designating nonprocreative acts as 'crimes against nature').

(Ertman, 2010: 23)

Arguing along a similar line of reasoning, Hoeyer (2009: 245) proposes that when the "logic of the free market" is introduced into exchanges, the result is neither a classic open market (the "bazaar"), nor "public health administration," but becomes more of a hybrid form comprising many different elements. As the exchange and trade of human biological material is always embedded in "moral reasoning," there is always some anxiety involved when such materials are traded as commodities (ibid.: 247). Hoeyer (ibid.) therefore believes that the "profanation" of sacred human biological materials and embryos and babies is less of a risk than critics contend:

'Humanness' … is in this case not an inert and stable quality threatened by a universal phenomenon known as 'the market,' but a product of material entities moving back and forth between the two semantic domains: 'personhood' and 'market.'

(Hoeyer, 2009: 245)

Hoeyer views the concepts of humanness and markets as co-produced, thus enabling specific exchange systems.

Ertman's (2010) argument in favor of markets for gametes and embryos does not ignore or trivialize the criticism of markets. For instance, in the case of egg donation, riddled by cases of women in e.g., Ukraine being encouraged to donate substantial amounts of their ova for economic compensation, there are strong reasons to be concerned about how to protect female donors. In this case, Ertman (ibid.) believes the negative consequences of paternalism – an effective ban on egg donation – are larger than the risks involved in creating a market for ova:

> Women as donors are more likely to suffer from objectification because their status as full citizens and legal subjects is relatively recent and, moreover, according to some accounts, remains incomplete. This law might worry if egg sales risked turning women into egg factories, or if they lacked the power to fully consent to the transactions. However, the dangers of paternalism seem to outweigh the benefits of protectionism in the prior instance.
>
> (Ertman, 2010: 32)

In fact, Ertman (2010: 33) argues that the egg donation process, including a hormone therapy and the unpleasant egg retrieval activities, justifies marketization. All this work and the physical experience of egg donation cannot be based on altruism alone but should also involve economic compensation.

In the case of sperm donations, Ertman (2010) sees few if any credible arguments against a market for sperm. In the case of embryos, things do become more complicated, though. This is due to the fact that this biological resource transgresses the "cultural dividing between people, which are not for sale, and things, which generally are" (Ertman, 2010: 33). In this view, embryos are certainly not "persons," yet they are not things but something in between that needs to be legally defined. Following her line of reasoning, Ertman (ibid.: 36) nevertheless suggests that embryos could be subject to "controlled commodification" similar to that of "pharmaceutical drugs."

Ertman's (2010) defense of markets for reproductive materials is by and large based on a critique of the majority's claim to speak on behalf of "nature," or "God," or any other factual or desired condition that should be fulfilled to qualify parents as being illegitimate or at least violating the statutes of Millian liberalism. "Market mechanisms present a different moral vision, which gives priority to liberty and innovation, rather than to tradition and divine or biological mandates," Ertman (ibid.: 23) summarizes her argument. The principal critique against markets for human reproductive materials, the concern for exploitation and a preference for what Ertman (ibid.) calls paternalism, can effectively be counteracted by legislation and its enforcement by competent professional regulatory agencies.

Krawiec (2010) takes a less ideological view and emphasizes the "externalities" of the market for babies, at the same time as she recognizes that today, this is a "three-billion-dollar industry" in the U.S. (ibid.: 42). In Krawiec's (ibid.: 48) view, the market is today biased and "a wide variety of fertility specialists, agents, brokers, facilitators, lawyers, and other middlemen" – what Krawiec (ibid.) refers to as *baby market intermediaries* – can therefore "legally profit handsomely" from the baby market. In this view, it is not so much a matter of articulating arguments in favor of or against a market for babies as it is a matter of securing its efficiency and a more equal distribution of the finance capital generated. Krawiec (2010) is concerned that what she refers to as *baby market competitors* have weak negotiation possibilities vis-à-vis the baby market intermediaries:

> Not coincidentally, baby market intermediaries have also agitated actively for legal and industry restrictions that impede the ability of birth parents, gestational surrogates, and egg donors (hereinafter called *baby market competitors*) – quite literally, the mom-and-pop producers in this industry – from collecting the market clearing price for their services, thus reducing competition and capping the price of their required inputs. Not surprisingly, then, supply in these sectors of the baby market frequently falls far short of demand.
>
> (Krawiec, 2010: 48)

To balance the interest between different baby market actors, Krawiec (2010: 50) suggests that a ban on "baby selling that prevents compensation to birth parents" would only give the baby market intermediaries a "[f]ree reign in setting placement fees and other expenses, make independent entry into the baby market less attractive for many baby market competitors, thus restricting market entry." A ban on markets for babies would de facto give monopoly licenses to the baby market intermediaries at the expense of both clients (i.e., would-be parents seeking assistance) and the baby market competitors. This would lead to, Krawiec (ibid.) says, (1) "inefficiently low supply and high consumer prices," and (2) "distributional concerns stemming from the distorted division of profits between baby market intermediaries and competitors." In addition to the efficiency and equal economic compensation arguments, Krawiec (ibid.: 52) rejects "grand normative statements about sacred values" commonly advanced to object to functional markets for babies and claims that such normative and moral declarations accomplish little more than to impede market transactions.

Spar (2010), in turn, objects to the view advanced by Landes and Posner (1978) and argues that children and reproductive materials cannot legitimately be examined as any commodity available on an open market. The market is not, as opposed to the neoclassical economic theory view, a neutral and superior mechanism for mediating interests and accommodating publicly available information, and consequently it cannot be treated as what effectively would handle issues derived from the clinical possibilities in assisted reproduction. "[M]arkets, we are tempted to respond, have nothing to do with reproductive freedom," Spar (2010: 177) says. She continues to argue that markets are not "inherently defined by a commitment to any set of rights," but when they work at their best, markets "encompass an intricate bundle of rules, norms, and traditions, all of which are directed at the dual pursuit of efficiency and profit maximization" (ibid.).

Unfortunately, markets have limited abilities to effectively take into consideration complex societal goals like "justice" or "equity" – there is, in short, Spar (2010: 177) claims, "no reason to suspect that markets will naturally produce these auxiliary benefits." This view is a much more delicate and nuanced account of the market and its functioning than that of Landes and Posner (1978) putting blind faith in the market as what would be able to solve a range of social issues and concerns. Such social issues and concerns includes abortion rates, and Landes and Posner (1978) formulate a proposition that assumes that a pregnancy and the delivery of a baby – and not least the separation of the mother of birth and her baby – would be a costless procedure devoid of both social stigma and "emotional work" on the part of the mother. If only unplanned pregnancies would be accompanied by the possibilities for economic compensation, more babies would be born, Landes and Posner (1978) predict, ignoring entirely that pregnancies are part of the human condition and deeply embedded in local cultures and institutional conditions rather than being some kind of paid-for service in a reproductive market.

In contrast, Spar (2010: 179) writes, "[r]eproduction is neither a public good (at least, in the customary economic use of that term) nor a common pool resource. Instead, reproduction is an innately *private* good." However, this line of argument does not lead Spar (2010: 1987) to finally reject the idea of markets for babies and reproductive materials and services, but she advocates a market that combines "commercial forces" and "government regulation" to protect reproductive rights. That is, no free-market solution as proposed by Landes and Posner (1978) would be able to fulfill the social needs and the demands for reasonable economic equality in terms of how the economic benefits are distributed among the actors participating in market transactions.

Yet another concern raised against forms of baby markets are that they would restore and reproduce racial and ethnic kinship that otherwise is counteracted by civil rights legislation. For instance, Goodwin (2010) examines the U.S. adoption market and notices some conspicuous forms of what is perhaps most appropriately described as racism in its classical form. In the U.S., couples may spend up to fifty thousand dollars to adopt a healthy white infant, whereas black babies are adopted for "as little as four thousand dollars" (ibid.: 5). In addition, an adoption of a black baby can be "facilitated in less than three weeks" (ibid.: 8), a substantially shorter period than for white babies. This pricing of babies may, however, reflect the "supply and demand" of babies of different colors in e.g., the case of if there are fewer black couples adopting from a larger stock of black babies, but it is complicated to explain some of the preferences articulated among e.g., women adopting a baby. For instance, whereas 86.4 percent of black women would accept a white child, the comparative figure for white women would be 72.5 percent. More noteworthy still, "more women expressed a preference for adopting a child with severe physical or mental disabilities than a preference for adopting a black child" (ibid.: 8). This racial discrimination is indicative of the higher degree of risk that black infants and children are exposed to in American society. For instance, 67 percent of all children living in foster care families are children of color (ibid.: 10). Such racial and ethnic beliefs and preferences cannot be effectively moderated by baby markets, but market protagonists such as Ertman (2010) would object that markets would not leverage these (undesirable) social beliefs, and nor can one expect markets to solve all social concerns. Instead, markets provide a set of mechanisms that enables privacy and secure individual rights from the majority's moral.

Taken together, the presence of ART in contemporary society and the possibilities these new technologies enable both provides a number of solutions to perceived problems but also create a new set of problems and challenges. While ART enables sub-fertile couples and single women to become parents, the very success of this new therapy creates a demand for gametes, which in turn create markets (as in the case of the U.S.) or pseudo-markets or hybrid markets (in the case of Sweden) for egg and sperm. As soon as there is locus for the trading of such reproductive materials, there will also be criticism against this trade. As for instance Almeling (2011) details in her ethnography of Californian egg and sperm donors, men and women are treating their participation in this market entirely differently (to be further discussed in Chapter 2) where, for instance, men took a more lighthearted view of their donations, joking about having "many children" and treating the economic compensation in terms of a salary. In contrast, the female donors were encouraged to think of their participation in egg donation as a form of gift-giving and treated their pay as a "compensation" (indicating a loss of something that can never be properly returned), and they were "certainly not mothers" (ibid.: 149). While sperm donation was surrounded by joking – "Making money never felt so good!", one ad at Craigslist declared – female egg donation was associated with a more solemn and serious attitude.

Donating egg cells undoubtedly is more of an ordeal for the female donor than it is for the male donor, but Almeling's (2011) study suggests that social and cultural beliefs surrounding female reproduction and sexuality, in many cases filtered through centuries of paternalism, is reflected in how egg donors are treated in the egg agencies. If nothing else, female donors are expected to express a great deal of empathy with sub-fertile couples and fellow women.

Innovations and the role of technoscience

It is widely believed that innovations are the mechanism that reproduce and invigorate the capitalist economic system (e.g., Solow, 1957). While neoclassical economic theory treated innovation as a relatively marginal phenomenon, the Austrian School of Economics scholar Joseph Schumpeter is generally advanced as the first major economist to fully recognize the role of innovations in the economy, even though Schumpeter himself made references to e.g., the work of the Austrian economist Eugen Böhm-Bawerk. Schumpeter (1942) speaks of innovations as "gales of creative destruction," which simultaneously create new opportunities, technical as well as economic and social, and actively destroys previous technologies. In Schumpeter's view, the capitalist economic system is characterized by this ceaseless process of creation and destruction, leading to more advanced technologies and more differentiated services.

In this context, innovation is defined in accordance with Crossan and Apaydin's (2010: 1155) four-partite definition, including (1) "Production or adoption, assimilation, and exploitation of a value-added novelty in economic and social spheres," (2) "Renewal and enlargement of products, services, and markets," (3) "Development of new methods of production," and (4) "establishment of new management systems" (ibid.: 1155. Original emphasis omitted). This is an all-encompassing definition, including both innovation in terms of new commodities and services and in terms of new production systems and managerial practices. That is, innovations can be both studied as *output* (e.g., commodities) and *processes* (new practices for reducing costs or increasing the value added).

In many cases, innovations are produced and brought to a market within a specific institutional setting or field (e.g., an industry, a technological domain), and therefore it is complicated to fully separate the innovation work located *inside* the firm and the activities taking place *outside* of the firm as this line of demarcation between the inside and the outside becomes porous and permeable. Cockburn and Stern (2010) speak of *innovation systems* as a concept that recognizes that innovations in many cases, if not most, are developed in the intersection between companies, universities, and industries, i.e., that innovation is more "open" than "closed" (see e.g., Chesbrough, 2003). "An innovation system consists of the interrelated and interdependent web of institutions and entities that contribute to the exploration, development, commercialization and diffusion of new knowledge and technology," Cockburn and Stern (2010: 9) write. Not least in the field of biomedical innovation and what Davey et al. (2011: 808) speak of as *health innovations*, there are intimate and close relationships and exchanges between companies, universities, institutes, and innovation system agencies, which all testify to the need to take an innovation system perspective on health innovations. In this specific institutional and economic setting, health innovations are defined accordingly:

> Health innovation consists of complex bundles of new medical technologies and clinical services emerging from a highly distributed competence base. Health innovation systems are driven by the combination of institutionally bound interactions or 'gateways' of innovation and history-dependent trajectories of change often referred to as pathways of innovation.
>
> (Davey et al., 2011: 808)

In the specific field of health innovations being examined in this volume, yet another analytical term needs to be introduced to accommodate the scientific complexities of reproductive medicine and assisted reproduction technologies.

The concept of technoscience was first introduced by the French philosopher of technology Gaston Bachelard and popularized by Jean-François Lyotard (1984) in his influential *La condition postmoderne* and the work of actor-network theorists including Bruno Latour and Michel Callon. Technoscience is a hybrid term, merging *technology* and *science* to underline that these are two mutually constitutive human resources and accomplishments; no technology without scientific thinking, and no science without the aid of advanced technologies for producing, recording, visualizing, storing, and computing data. As many studies of technoscientific practices in either the laboratory setting or in fieldwork demonstrates, in the era of late-modern technoscience, nature is no longer what is "described" or "discovered" but instead it is created, mimicked, and manipulated, for instance in the form of experimental systems (e.g., genetically modified animals, yeast cell lines) and in the creation of epistemic objects (genomic sequences, bacteria, proteins, etc.) (Rheinberger, 1997, 2010). This procedure is accentuated in what Taylor (2005: 743) names the *biomedical technosciences*, defined in somewhat opaque terms as "[t]hose rapidly emerging projects of knowledge-production and intervention that are both intensively focused on delineating the (universal) body and increasingly imposed on actual, particular bodies and the subjects who inhabit them." Technoscience no longer examines nature as a "brute fact," but recreate elements of nature in the laboratory that can be controlled and disciplined to enable an examination under stable and predictable conditions.

> The conjunction of technics, science, and this new mobility of capital signals the opening of a future that is to be systematically explored through experimentation. As science has become technoscience it *describes* the real less and less, and is indeed what increasingly radically destabilizes it. Technical science no longer depicts what *is* (the law of life): it *creates* a new reality; it is a science of becoming.
>
> (Stiegler, 2011: 191)

Somewhat paradoxically, at least in the field of advanced biomedical technosciences, technoscientific research work is firmly confined to the laboratory setting where many parameters can be kept under strict control, and yet technoscientific authority expands well beyond this narrow domain as it effectively enrolls and mobilizes a variety of stakeholders and actors (Latour, 1988, 1995):

> Technoscience goes beyond the boundaries of the laboratories, even though the laboratory is an essential site for technoscientific production. Technoscience is equally produced in the deliberations and actions of policymakers (state and nonstate), market actors, activists (whether opposed to technoscience or fighting it for its acceleration or intensification), consumers of various sorts, editors of scientific journals, and patients … Technoscience is always already many things – a collection of institutions, normative structures, practices, and ideologies.
>
> (Sunder Rajan, 2012: 17)

As a consequence of this enfolding of technoscientific work and the various policy, regulatory, financial, etc., work it generates, "human action and technoscience are co-constitutive, thereby refuting technoscientific determinisms," Clarke et al. (2003: 165) say. This is an important point being raised by Sunder

Rajan (2012) and Clarke et al. (2003) as there are today anxieties regarding where technoscience and medical technoscience in particular may take us and how it opens up new possibilities for manipulating "the innermost secrets of life" (see e.g., Habermas, 2003). This anxiety may encourage a view of technoscience as a form of monolithic machinery capable of operating outside of a wider institutional framework and creating its own momentum outside of human influence. Such concerns may be mediated by the insight that technoscience remains in the hands of humans, and that the movement from the laboratory to wider society demands much work and many agreements.

The site of biomedical technoscience: universities as engines of economic growth

As biomedical technoscience has advanced its positions since the 1970s, the university has become a central site for the research work that propels the innovation work in e.g., the pharmaceutical and biotechnology industries. The biomedical technosciences is a combination of two academic disciplines demonstrating their own historical pathways: chemistry and biology. Chemistry was one of the first academic disciplines to become fully professionalized during the nineteenth century (Bensaude-Vincent and Stengers, 1996). In first Prussia and thereafter in a number of German states, the medieval university system was reformed from within by skilled and visionary bureaucrats and state functionaries in the first half of the nineteenth century. After 1801, economic reforms in Prussia included guild restrictions, land reforms, labor reforms, and changes in the university system (Lenoir, 1998: 22). In the period 1840–1870, a new "research ethos" was established in the German universities, focusing on performance and competition between German states to develop the best university system.

Chemistry was the academic discipline that was actively encouraged at an early stage to collaborate with industry to create joint benefits and interests. In both Germany and Sweden, chemistry was professionalized and developed in tandem with the mining industry and thus became the first university discipline in the modern sense of the term. In France, in contrast, the discipline remained a "science of amateurs," still relying on experimental demonstrations in salons or public and private courses (Bensaude-Vincent and Stengers, 1996: 64). Chemistry was also the first discipline for which an international congress of specialists was organized, at Karlsruhe in 1860 (ibid.: 95). The Prussian initiative to create a university system that added to the competitiveness or innovativeness of industry was thus very successful, and there were many examples of fruitful and long-standing collaborations across the industry–university boundaries, including for instance close collaborations between Farbwerke Hoechts and Robert Koch's research laboratory (Lenoir, 1998: 25). In other words, through thoughtful reforms in the university system, chemistry was constituted as an academic discipline from within the university system.

The other disciplinary branch of biomedical technoscience, biology and physicology, demonstrates an entirely different trajectory. While medicine has always been a domain of prestige and authority from the ancient period, it was not until the development of Edward Jenner's smallpox vaccine in 1798 that there is any evidence of any efficient therapy developed in clinical medicine (Collins, 1979: 139). Instead, medicine in the classical period was very much a source of jokes as medical doctors were by and large unable to cure their patients. Voltaire, for instance, claimed that "the art of the medical profession" consisted of the capacity to amuse the patient "as long as it takes nature to cure him or her" (cited in Blech, 2006: ix). Incompetent and pretentious physicians also feature in no less than four of Molière's comedies, indicating the public's low esteem of the profession. Rather than being a proper scientific discipline and practice, physicians were competing with "wise women, herbalists, good Samaritans, midwives, itinerant drug peddlers, ladies of the manor, mountebanks, and quacks" over discretionary jurisdiction in the domain of illness and health (Bynum, 1994: 2).

However, after the French revolution things changed swiftly. In 1794, "the *annus mirabilis* of medicine" in Bynum's (1994: 26) account, the French authorities decided to open *Écoles de Santé* in a number of French cities including Strasbourg, Montpellier, and Paris. While medicine had been taught in e.g., Sorbonne since the medieval period, the Paris faculty was notoriously conservative and had opposed the work of Vesalius in the sixteenth century, Harvey in the seventeenth, and remained one of the last bastions of the ancient doctrine of Galenism (ibid.). This stronghold of ancient teachings was not fertile ground for a theoretical and practical discipline. Fortunately, in this period experimentalists such as Marie François Xavier Bichat (1771–1802), originally trained as a surgeon (ibid.: 31), one of the few medical specialisms where there was a widespread clinical experience enabled by the service of surgeons in the armies, developed new experimental methods (Haigh, 1984). By the mid-nineteenth century a new generation of empirically oriented researchers including Claude Bernard, trained in the new open *Écoles de Santé* tradition of thinking, had advanced medicine as an experimental and empirical scientific discipline. In 1865, Claude Bernard published his seminal *An introduction to the study of experimental medicine*, regarded as a standard work for a long period of time.

While medicine had to shake off the conservatism of the medieval university system to develop its own methodologies and its own institutions – the medical school built in close proximity to the large public hospitals, providing a steady inflow of patients – the adjacent academic discipline of biology did not gain momentum until the late nineteenth century. As detailed by Evelyn Fox Keller (2000, 2002), biology was the last of the modern science disciplines to consolidate itself. While chemistry proved its practical utility in the nineteenth century and physics had its golden age in the 1880–1930 period including the work of a series of famed physicists including Konrad Lorenz, Albert Einstein, and Werner von Heisenberg – all household names denoting brilliance and genius – biology was emerging as a scandalous scholarly pursuit as the Christian community was enraged by Charles Darwin's claim in his *The Origin of Species* (1857) that humans were not created by God as prescribed in *Genesis* but rather descended from primates through processes of mutation, adaptation, and selection over thousands of millennia.

Such un-Godly claims could not be tolerated and to this day Darwinism remains disputed by e.g., the American Christian right. It was arguably not until Francis Crick and James Watson's "discovery" of the double helix structure of DNA, the principal hereditary material of biological organisms, that experimental and theoretical biology could finally claim the authority and legitimacy that were granted the disciplines of chemistry, physics, and medicine much earlier. On the other hand, in the post-World War II period, and after 1980 in particular, biology as a science has entrenched the position as the jewel in the crown of the sciences, enabling an entirely new understanding of biological systems at the molecular, cellular, and organ levels and thus creating possibilities for new clinical practices and therapies prolonging human lives and reducing pain and suffering for millions of human beings on a daily basis.

While the developmental paths of the sciences has been both crooked and straight, there is today a wide acclaim of the sciences and their locus, the universities, as being "economic engines" as scientific know-how can be commercially exploited (Berman, 2012). Such hopes and expectations are commonly rooted in the increased level of patenting being observed in e.g., the U.S. university system since the mid-1960s, a phenomenon that led to the Bayh-Dole Act of 1980 granting universities the right to patent its publicly funded research results (Mowery, 2009: 37). In addition, the new role of the universities is closely bound up with the relative decline in federal research funding in the military sector and the growth of biomedical and life science research funding. In 1959, the defense-related share of federal R&D spending peaked at the whopping level of 85 percent. Thereafter it declined somewhat but in the Reagan era, characterized by a large budget deficit and high levels of military spending, it was back at a 70 percent level. In 1999, after the fall of the iron curtain and the decline of what many Americans treated as "the communist threat," the low point of 54 percent of defense-related R&D in the federal budget was reported (ibid.: 30). The declining defense-related research work opened up for life sciences and biomedical research (ibid.: 30), benefitting the universities providing such research competencies and research skills. In the 1980s and 1990s, the income from licensing fees derived from previous successful research work and research collaborations with industry accounted for 66 to 85 percent of the gross licensing revenues of many academic institutions (ibid.: 39). Life science research work seemed to pay off quite well.

The firm belief in the universities as the engines of economic growth also coincides with the decline of the productivity of the internal or in-house R&D departments in large organizations. Block and Keller (2009) report that there are comparatively fewer innovations, measured in terms of patenting activity produced in the Standard & Poor 500 companies, in the U.S. today. In addition, fewer scientists are employed in these large firms as they have increasingly outsourced and off-shored their R&D activities to smaller companies or to countries with lower factor costs. "In 1971, 7.6% of all R&D scientists and engineers working, or 28,000 individuals were employed by firms by fewer than 10,000 employees. By 2004, this percentage had risen to 32%, while the actual number had grown to 365,000," Block and Keller (2009: 470) report. As a consequence of this decline of the integrated and self-enclosed R&D department, "university-based science efforts" are more closely linked to industry, and "government agencies are playing an increasingly central role in managing and facilitating the process of technological development" (Block and Keller, 2009: 463). In other words, R&D and innovation work are today organized in a network-based structure (see e.g., Nielsen, 2012; Paruchuri, 2010; Whittington, Owen-Smith, and Powell, 2009; Powell et al., 2005; Owen-Smith and Powell, 2004):

> [T]he declining centrality of the largest corporations to the innovation process in the US, the growing importance of inter-organizational collaboration and small start-up firms in the innovation process. And the expanded role of public sector institutions as both participants in and funders of innovation processes.
>
> (Block and Keller, 2009: 475)

One of the theoretical and practical implications is that the strong belief in markets as the principal and superior mechanism for regulating and pricing innovative capacities cannot be assumed to be adequate as the public sector funding and the intermediary role of public sector organization (see e.g., Obstfeld, 2005) play a decisive role in advancing and supporting the new life science based economy – the bioeconomy. Block and Keller's (2009: 476) findings thus "[c]ontradict the market fundamentalist ideology that celebrates private enterprise and denigrades the public sector." Block and Keller's (2009) research findings have many implications for innovation policy and the practical work to finance and support life science innovations, not least to secure an adequate supply of venture capital (Styhre, 2015), but it also, similar to Berman's (2012) account, emphasizes the role of the research university as an important node in both local, regional, and international innovation networks. After 1980 and the enactment of the Bayh-Dole Act – arguably more a consequence than a driver of university patenting activity (Mirowski, 2011: 117) – universities were given a new role, not entirely different from the one conceived by the Prussian state officials in the first half of the nineteenth century, as what both bridges and bonds various actors in network-based innovative activities and provides systematic research findings that can become subject to venturing and commercialization.

Outline of the book

This volume is structured into eight chapters and divided into this introduction chapter, Part I, Theoretical perspectives, Part II, Empirical studies, and Part III, Institutionalizing ART. The first part of the volume includes two chapters: Chapter 2 reviews the institutional theory literature and pays specific attention to the concept of agency within this theoretical framework that otherwise emphasizes various forms, convergences and isomorphisms in e.g., industries and professional fields. Chapter 3 examines the literature on reproductive therapies and the market for such services. In Part II of the volume, the empirical material is presented. This part of the book is separated into a methodology chapter and three elementary institutional work processes, namely the creation of institutions (Chapter 5), the maintenance of institutions (Chapter 6) and the disrupting of institutions (Chapter 7). These three chapters highlight different practices and activities among the various groups that are involved in the ART field. The final part of the book consists of one single chapter, summarizing the key research findings and discussing the theoretical and practical implications derived from the empirical material. Discussing the institutional work of the various actors engaging in shaping and informing the field as a way to create "reproductive futures," the volume concludes that human reproduction and human fertility is by no means a fixed and stable practice or resource but novel scientific procedures, new social norms and ethics, and regulatory regimes are constantly influencing and shaping how human fertility is to be understood and discussed. In other words, the reproductive future of mankind is open for new ideas and new practices, and a democratization of ART would be welcome, no longer benefitting only the richest economic groups in a few welfare states but becoming accessible for a wider set of stakeholders, also in the less economically developed parts of the world.

Summary and conclusion

This introductory chapter has discussed how reproductive medicine has gradually moved from being a research work activity in universities and research institutes, and has gradually become entrenched as a clinical practice, now being offered on a market for reproductive services. In many ways, the field of reproductive medicine has been one of the most successful life science projects in terms of its ability to directly influence everyday life for millions of people – in the Western part of the world, where IVF is available for a larger share of the population, one child out of 30 is today born on the basis of assisted reproduction – but also in terms of changing the entire attitude towards human fertility and parenting. Now, the failure to become parents is no longer simply understood as a cruel twist of fate but becomes a health care concern, part of what is widely addressed as reproductive health. However, this success comes with the cost of determining politically or through market transactions whether reproductive health care services should be part of the welfare state provisions or if it should be provided by market-based actors. The debate regarding the advantages of the two systems includes a variety of perspectives, ranging from free market advocacy, assuming that markets are simply the more efficient mechanism for pricing and lowering the costs for such services, to the argument that the planned system of the public health care system would easily discredit and marginalize minorities' (e.g., single women, lesbian couples, gay men) interests. In addition, some commentators reject market-based solutions altogether on the basis that human reproduction is no standardized commodity that can lend itself to market pricing mechanisms. Regardless of the perspective taken, the blending of market thinking and human reproduction creates a sense of uneasiness that arguably does not reside in the capacity for rational human thinking but is derived from the tint of emotionality that human reproduction induces. In other words, parenting and the birth of children are not effortlessly apprehended by the market transaction vocabulary and the economic reasoning that pertains to other services and commodities.

Part I

Theoretical perspectives

2 Institutional theory and the concept of agency

Introduction

In what may be called classic organization theory being developed the first two decades after World War II, organizations were increasingly treated as fundamentally open to their environment and responsive to external changes. Parsons (1956) defined organizations on the basis of his general structural theory as a "social system" that is characterized by its "orientation to the attainment of a specific goal" (ibid.: 64. Original emphasis omitted). In addition, Parsons (ibid.: 64) defines "the attainment of a goal" as the "*relation* between a system" and "the relevant parts of the external situation in which [the system, i.e., the organizations] acts or operates." This most formalistic definition, not exactly an impressive piece of academic writing in terms of crisp clarity, by and large summarized Philip Selznick's portrayal of organizations in his seminal *TVA and the grassroots* (1949) as being socially embedded in wider environments: "No organization subsists in a vacuum. Large or small, it must pay some heed to the consequences of its own activities (and even existence) for other groups and forces in the community" (Selznick, 1949: 10). In 1966, Katz and Kahn (1966) published the first major work that would later be treated as a body of texts that was referred to as *contingency theory*. Also in contingency theory, the organization's openness to its milieu was emphasized. For Katz and Kahn (ibid.: 17), organizations are "flagrantly open systems," wherein there are continuously transactions being made between "the organization and its environment." Katz and Kahn (ibid.: 47) were faithful to the functionalist systems theory view developed by Parsons, saying that organizations are composed of a set of interrelated, structural systems:

(1) Organizations possess a *maintenance* structure as well as *production* and *production-supportive* structures ... (2) organizations have an *elaborated formal role pattern* in which a division of labor results in a functional specificity of roles ... (3) There is a *clear authority structure* in the organization which reflects the way in which the control and managerial function is exercised. (4) As part of the managerial structure there are multi-developed regulatory mechanisms and *adaptive structures* ... (5) There is an

explicit formulation of *ideology* to provide systems norms which buttress the authority structure.

(Katz and Kahn, 1966: 47)

The most well-known contingency theory work (James Thompson's [1967] *Organizations in Action* being the other work), Paul R. Lawrence and Jay W. Lorsch's *Organization and Environment* (1967) further developed the open-system view of organization but added the idea that an organization's internal structure and degree of differentiation was more or less mirroring the diversity of the environment wherein the organization operates: "The most successful organizations tended to maintain states of differentiation and integration consistent with the diversity of the part of the environment and the required interdependence of the parts" (Lawrence and Lorsch, 1967: 134). The degree of formalization was therefore treated by contingency theorists as a function of the perceived unpredictability and uncertainty of the environment: "The more unpredictable and uncertain the parts of the environment, the lower in the organizational hierarchy this tends to be" (ibid.: 157–158). In addition, the more differentiated the internal structure, the more difficult the integration of the parts, and therefore, organizations operating in dynamic, changeable, and unpredictable milieus are more complicated to manage as environmental complexities mirror the formal organization. Thompson (1967) spoke about this organization–environment nexus in terms of *homeostasis* or *self-stabilization*, a form of spontaneous or natural equilibrium that regulated and governs "[t]he necessary relationships among parts and keeps the system viable in the face of disturbances stemming from the environment" (ibid.: 7).

This locates managers in the precarious position where they on the one hand are expected to believe in rational methods for managing the activities and assessing performance and outcomes, but where, on the other hand, they have to anticipate and cope with a series of uncertainties and contingencies. This makes managerial work – "the process of administration," in Thompson's (1967) vocabulary – a process essentially concerned with the handling of forms of uncertainty in order to maintain the *homeostasis*:

> The process of administration may be thought of as providing boundaries within which organizational rationality becomes possible. In this view administration is the process of copying with uncertainty, but it is not merely the defensive absorption of blockage of uncertainty. Administration includes a more aggressive co-alignment aspect which keeps the organization at the nexus of several necessary streams of action.
>
> (Thompson, 1967: 162)

Contingency theory's modified version of Parsonian systems theory, recognizing the functional differentiation of the organizational structure, was very influential in the 1960s and 1970s, but by the end of the 1970s, there were at least two distinct theoretical contributions further developing the idea of organizations as open systems (Katz and Kahn, 1966) or natural systems (Thompson, 1967). First, the resource-dependency theory advocated by Pfeffer and Salancik (1978) recognized the environment's influence on organization structure but claimed that this influence was partial and indirect rather than determinate: "Organizations are only loosely coupled with the environment," Pfeffer and Salacik (ibid.: 227) stated. They continued: "The fact that environmental impacts are felt only imperfectly provides the organization with some discretion, as well as the capability to act across time horizons longer than the time it takes for environments to change" (ibid.: 13). At the same time, organizations are indisputably dependent on their environment to secure access to vital resources and for creating the legitimacy needed to ensure long-term survival of the firm – a key issue for a variety of organization theory schools.

While demonstrating many connections with contingency theory, resource-dependency is widely recognized as a free-standing contribution to organization theory. In contrast, Meyer and Rowan's (1977) seminal work and arguably the starting point for neoinstitutional theory took its key terms from the works of Philip Selznick and other institutional theorists in the disciplines of e.g., sociology, anthropology, and economics (e.g., the work of Thorstein Veblen). Despite recognizing such historical roots, the article of Meyer and Rowan (ibid.) in many ways served to rearticulate and re-popularize the ideas of Parsons and the contingency theorists but expressed in a less formalist vocabulary. Meyer and Rowan (ibid.: 340) speak of "formal organizations" as "systems of coordinated and controlled activities that arise when work is embedded in complex networks of technical relations and boundary-spanning exchanges." Again, organizations are understood to operate at the nexus between internal differentiation and coordination (i.e., forms of managerial activities) and the environment.

In order to keep internal demands for efficiency and external demands for legitimacy, Meyer and Rowan (1977) strongly emphasize the role of loose couplings between formal structures and "institutional rules": "To maintain ceremonial conformity, organizations that reflect institutional rules tend to buffer their formal structures from the uncertainties of technical activities by becoming loosely coupled, building gaps between their formal structures and the actual work activities" (ibid.: 341). That is, in the operative vocabulary of Chris Argyris and Donald Schön (1978), there is a divergence between *espoused theories* (theories that are formally and officially endorsed) and *theories-in-use* (the actual practices of the organizations) in the organization. Such loose couplings between functional units and between practices officially acclaimed and practically implemented were recognized by contingency theorists, but the neoinstitutional analytical framework outlined by Meyer and Rowan (1977) was bolder in terms of questioning the Parsonian view of organizations as enclosed and functional social systems existing *sui generis*:

Quite beyond the environmental interrelations suggested in open-systems theories, institutional theories in their extreme forms define organizations as dramatic enactments of the rationalized myths pervading modern societies, rather than as units involved in exchange – no matter how complex – with their environments.

(Meyer and Rowan, 1977: 346)

Organizations are therefore no longer indisputable "facts" and ensembles of tangible resources and accompanying know-how but rather become "dramatic enactments" of the myths and ceremonies including the norm of rationality upon which modern managerial ideologies and practices rest. One of the consequences of this enactment of the organization – still today, radical in its recognition of symbolism and beliefs as constitutive elements of organization – is that institutionalized norms and practices may actively inhibit or intervene into the organization's "logic of efficiency," its pursuit to optimize its use of resources in its day-to-day operations and practices. According to Meyer and Rowan (1977: 355): "Categorical rules conflict with the logic of efficiency. Organizations often face the dilemma that activities celebrating institutionalized rules, although they count as virtuous ceremonial expenditures, are pure costs from the point of view of efficiency."

All these classic accounts of organization and its formal and informal structure, its differentiation, coordination and integration, assume that organization is a form of systemic arrangement characterized by its ceaseless response to environmental conditions and changes. In addition – and this is a key point in this context – these theoretical accounts of organization speak primarily about "super-individual" entities such as organizations, the environment, organization units, and so forth. Testifying to the analytical heritage of Talcott Parson's influential functionalist systems theory, there are few accounts of any actors or agency in this theoretical framework. Instead, organizations are anthropomorphized in their ghostlike ability to act and respond without any humans being involved and playing any significant roles. Organizations are thus understood as astral bodies in a solar system being kept in equilibrium, but otherwise operating on a cosmic level where human influence is nigh.

In order to counteract this "organization theory without agents," this chapter will examine how institutional theory has gradually "discovered" the role of actors and agency and how recent contributions in the new millennium has inscribed the human actor into the institutional theory perspective. In order to understand and examine how ART are being further developed and brought into the clinics and to the market, there is a need for both recognizing system-level changes and the changes in everyday work practices and work routines in specific communities and settings. In other words, this chapter will be dedicated to the analysis of how Parsonian systems theory, highly influential in the 1950s and 1960s, has gradually fallen from grace and been displaced by theories of practice representing an entirely different tradition within social theory. This analysis paves the way for the discussion about ART and the expansion of reproductive medicine in Chapter 3 and the presentation of the empirical material in Part II of this volume.

Operative definitions and epistemological positions

In order to proceed with the analysis of how agency has increasingly been recognized in organization theory more generally and in institutional theory more specifically, there is a need for a set of definitions. First of all, to draw an epistemological line of demarcation between neoclassical economic theory and economic sociology and its specialized branch of organization theory, we can follow Trigilia (2002) in his distinction between the economy as (1) an "institutionalized process," i.e., as a "system," and, (2) as the practice of "economizing." Trigilia (ibid.: 2. Original emphasis omitted) defines the former as "[a] body of activities which are usually carried out by members of a society in order to produce, distribute, and exchange goods and services." The latter is defined as "activities which involve the rational allocation of scarce resources in order to obtain the most from the means available" (ibid.: 2. Original emphasis omitted). For economic sociologists, Trigilia (ibid.: 3. Original emphasis omitted) writes, "economic activity is an institutionalized process." That is, the analysis of the economy must effectively accommodate the actor-structure problem inherent to all social science theory, the mutual recognition of both the structural and systemic nature of "the economy" and the forms of agency and possibilities for enterprising activities provided within this system. Still, the concept of institution is of key relevance here, being defined by Trigilia (ibid.: 4. Emphasis in the original) as "[a] *set of social norms which orient and regulate behavior and which are based on sanctions which seek to guarantee compliance on the part of the individual.*"

This definition of institutions needs to be anchored in the extensive literature on institutions and institutional theory. Parsons (1951: 39) defines an institution as "[a] complex of institutionalized roles integrated which is of strategic structural significance in the social system in question." In this functionalist systems theory view, institutions are "roles," but there is no account of from where these roles emerge in the first place. In the more "soft" and "cognitivistic" version of institutional theory represented by e.g., Émile Durkheim and anthropologist Mary Douglas, institutions are defined as "[a]ll the beliefs and all the modes of conduct instituted by the collectivity" (Durkheim, [1895] 1938: lxi). As a consequence, for Douglas (1986), the "entrenching" of an institution is "[a]n intellectual process as much as an economic and political one" (ibid.: 45). Douglas even goes so far to claim that institutions "think and feel" for human beings, help them perceive and to act in accordance with prescribed and sanctioned standard operation procedures: "Institutions systematically direct individual memory and channel our perception into forms compatible with the relations they authorize" (ibid.: 92). Not everyone would agree with this definition of institutions, making it a kind of Durkheimian *conscience collective* (Durkheim, 1895) and some shared, communal cognitive structure, but would rather favor a more restricted definition.

In this volume, the cognitive aspects of institutions are recognized insofar as they influence e.g., professional identities and roles and prescribe standard operation procedures in everyday work life activities, but they by no means determine the life world of organizational actors. Therefore, a more mainstream economic sociology view of institutions as being "shared rules," which can be laws or "collective understandings," held in place by "custom, explicit agreement, or tacit agreement" (Fligstein, 1996: 658), is followed. This definition opens up analytical differences between, for instance, law and regulatory frameworks and institutions, a key distinction when examining ART and reproductive medicine where legal and regulatory frameworks and ethical issues and recommendations are easily separated from what can be practically accomplished on the basis of technoscientific reproductive medicine and its clinical practices. This represents a moderate view of institutions as containing cognitive and social or cultural elements and as playing a role in constituting the economy and the organization.

In addition, in the analysis of ART and reproductive medicine, there is a need for a definition of the market. Fligstein (1996: 658) offers a useful definition: "*Markets* refer to situations in which some good or service is sold to customers for a price that is paid in money (a generalized medium of exchange)." Aspers (2010: 1) more specifically emphasizes the role of competition in setting the prices: "I define *market* as a social structure for the exchange of rights in which offers are evaluated and priced, and compete with one another." For Aspers (ibid.), markets cannot be defined outside of the economic term *competition*, being a concept denoting the process wherein actors jointly create possibilities and mechanisms for settling price disputes and making prices predictable and products and services commensurable over time. In the field of ART and assisted reproduction, prices are commonly negotiated and settled by various institutional actors and therefore the pricing process in this domain is by and large a heavily politicized and regulated process. When pricing what is essentially priceless (Zelizer, 1985) and what is part of intimate life (ibid.) – human reproduction – price-setting cannot be expected to occur through open-market bidding (e.g., auctions, see e.g., Velthuis, 2011: 180) without the loss of legitimacy in domains beset by strong norms and beliefs. Instead, the pricing of assisted reproduction services occurs on the basis of discussions in close-knit communities including representatives of clinics, public health care organizations, and regulatory bodies.

Law, politics, and governance in institutions

Institutional theorists have long recognized that legalization and regulatory frameworks actively influence organizations and determine how they structure their internal, functional departments and activities (Edelman, 1992; Sutton et al., 1994). As opposed to common sense thinking, predicting that laws prescribe what practices are unlawful, institutional theorists argue that laws tend to be quite imprecise and that they offer little direct advice or instructions on how to translate laws into organizational practices and managerial oversight (see e.g., Coates, 2007), and consequently laws have unintended consequences (Edelman, 1990). For instance, studying equal opportunities legislation and their implications for human resource management practices, Dobbin and Sutton (1998: 470) found that organizations created new offices "[n]ot because the law dictated that they do so but because the law did not tell them *what* to do." This finding supports the previous work of Baron, Dobbin and Jennings (1986), demonstrating that new personnel administration routines were developed in large firms when the government defined "high turnover" to be a problem to consider and properly handle, but that there were no direct compulsory rules regarding *how* to deal with the problem. As a consequence, Baron, Dobbin and Jennings (ibid.) show, the companies themselves were made responsible for how to organize their new personnel administration department, leading to a sharp increase in formal expertise in personnel administration:

> The number of personnel and labor relations professional in the United States increased from fewer than 30,000 in 1946 to 53,000 in 1950 and 93,000 in 1969 ... in percentage terms, the growth rate of the personnel profession far outstripped the growth rate of other professions ...
>
> (Baron, Dobbin and Jennings, 1986: 375)

Another case where new legislation and regulatory framework leads to organizational changes to accommodate such institutional shifts is Zorn's (2004) study of how changes in demands for financial reporting in the U.S., beginning with the Celler-Kefauver Act of 1950, led to the increase in the number of Chief Financial Officers within the top management team in stock-listed companies. Fligstein (1987, 1990) argued persuasively that the role of CFOs increased during the wave of hostile takeover bids in the 1980s, thus being indicative of the "power struggles" between proponents of a *managerial capitalism* regime dominated by managerial oversight and authority and an *investor capitalism* regime relying on finance market control of managers. As opposed to this explanation, Zorn (2004) argues that the regulatory changes date back to the 1950s, and that the new earnings-reporting requirements enacted after 1978 in particular, caused these changes: "Responding to the passage of the Celler-Kefauver Act in 1950, and changes, finance managers won the battle over who held the strategic key to the future, displacing experts in sales at the helm of the largest corporations," Zorn (ibid.: 349) summarizes.

Taken together, this literature examining the role of law and regulatory frameworks in determining and influencing organizational activities stresses not so much the market and competition as what structure organizations but the formal laws and regulations, not always straightforward or unambiguous, constitute the environment of organizations. This institutional theory view runs counter to both economic theory – in the most orthodox case treating law and regulations as unnecessary complications intervening into naturally efficient markets – but also violates what Dobbin and Sutton (1998: 472) speak about as American common sense thinking:

> Americans develop collective amnesia about the state's role in shaping private enterprises ... Americans subscribe to the theory that firms operate in a Hobbesian economic state of nature, in which behavior depends very much

on managerial initiative and markets and very little on political initiative and law.

(Dobbin and Sutton, 1998: 472)

As a consequence, law and regulations need to be recognized when studying how new fields of medicine are institutionalized and established. Theoretically speaking, how formal law is translated into various forms of governance will be examined below.

Governance, technologies of government, and governance devices

Miller and Rose (1990: 8), drawing on what Foucault speaks of as *governmentality*, introduce the concepts of *programs of government* and *technologies of government*. Programs of government are wider and more far-reaching political and economic objectives to govern societies and social systems, and *technologies of government* are the various tools, methods, and techniques developed to accomplish governance objectives. These technologies include techniques of notation and computation, calculative practices of examination and assessment, the invention of surveys and league tables, and the "inauguration of professional specialisms and vocabularies," etc., all aiming at instituting predictable and widely shared practices and routines for governance work. Miller and Rose (ibid.: 10–11) stress that government programs are ongoing, ceaseless pursuits encountering their own limitations en route. For instance,

> [T]echnologies produce unexpected problems, are utilized for their own ends by those who are supposed to merely operate them, are hampered by underfunding, professional rivalries, and the impossibility of producing technical conditions that would make them work – reliable statistics, efficient communication systems, clear lines of command, properly designed buildings, well framed regulations or whatever.

(Miller and Rose, 1990: 10–11)

Du Gay, Millo and Tuck (2012: 1085) speak of such technologies of government as *governance devices*, tools and resources that "transcend divisions between the actor and the device and create a new kind of agency – an assemblage." That is, Du Gay, Millo and Tuck (ibid.: 1085) suggest, governance devices cannot be seen as mere tools, completely devoid of agency but must be understood within a wider system of governance. This is also the contribution of Du Gay, Millo and Tuck (ibid.: 1085), that they do not equate governance devices with a set of tools or techniques, but that they are instead what Gilles Deleuze speaks of as *assemblages*, as "[c]lusters of people, machines, and institutionalized processes that operate interactively towards an organizationally defined goal."

Both Miller and Rose (1990) and Du Gay, Millo and Tuck (2012) draw on a continental philosophy tradition of thought (Foucault and Deleuze, respectively), making quite abstract statements about the nature of governance and the tools and procedures involved. In institutional theory, the concept of governance is less abstractly defined as corporate law, property rights, and forms of governance structures being implemented to secure that a variety of stakeholders are able to have their interests recognized and at least partially secured. The most important governance tool is corporate law, which defines "[t]he legal vehicles by which property rights are organized" (Fligstein and Choo, 2005: 63). Property rights, defined as "social relations that define who has claims on the profits of firms" (Fligstein, 1996: 658), are part of the governance system. In addition to property law, historically speaking, corporate law has always "performed a balancing act with management discretion and shareholder power," Bratton and Wachter (2010: 659) argue, pointing at the dual role of corporate law to both secure the interests of various stakeholders and to create possibilities for efficient markets. Proponents of finance market-based control of managerial effectiveness, declaring that shareholder value creation is not only the superior but also the only legitimate governance mechanism to discipline managers and to curb managerial malfeasance, criticize corporate law for creating unnecessary complications and therefore, by implication, justifying higher transaction and agency costs (see e.g., Rock, 2013: 1986). In this case, corporate law is assessed in terms of strict efficiency criteria at the expense of other legal objectives, such as economic stability, stakeholder interests, and the question of externalities created in the corporate system. In advancing such criticism, shareholder value protagonists turn a blind eye to the historical record of corporate law, Roy (1997: 174) suggests: "The changes created by corporate law were not necessarily conducive to greater efficiency, technological development, or managerial effectiveness. The explanations of the corporate revolution that focuses on technological adaptation, managerial efficiency, or economic power miss part of the story." In addition, the governance system or what Peet (2011: 386) speaks of as a *policy regime* – a systematic approach to policy formation, by a set of government or governance institutions – includes labor law and other forms of legal and regulatory frameworks that constitute the environment of an organization.

The so-called corporate governance literature has engaged in quite extensive comparative studies between nations, regions, and economies to determine what governance system or policy regimes are the most likely to produce economic growth and well-being. The result seems to be mixed, with no one-best-way-solution to be found. Instead, stability, predictability, and a low degree of opportunistic behavior appear to be a winning recipe, Fligstein and Choo (2005) argue:

> [H]aving well-defined property rights that grant ownership of profits to individuals are generally positive for economic growth. [The literature] also shows that well-developed financial institutions offer would be entrepreneurs the opportunity to grow new firms ... Finally, there is little evidence that labor laws that provide more extensive worker rights and welfare provisions inhibit economic growth.
>
> (Fligstein and Choo, 2005: 75–76)

That is, there is no evidence of the so-called liberal market economies (e.g., the U.S. and the U.K.) creating higher economic growth than so-called embedded liberalism economies, including Germany and the Scandinavian countries. In addition, the critique of labor unions as what inhibits economic growth through making unwarranted claims on behalf of their members or otherwise to encourage labor market reforms is not substantiated as union activity show limited effects on economic growth. Therefore, various governance systems appear to have their own specific advantages, benefit and risks, but it is complicated to prescribe one best model on the basis of economic data.

Despite this "diversity of governance systems view," the very idea of regimes of governance as what regulates and balances the interests of various stakeholders' interests opens up for politics and power, the home-turf of sociologists and critical theory scholars. Such a view invites a dual perspective on organizations, where institutions are, on the one hand, to be understood from a *contractarian* perspective where socially unbound individuals make agreement, legal or "psychological," and from a *political*, *social*, and *cultural* perspective wherein individuals' goals, objectives and strategies and tactics to accomplish these goals are taken into account. Owen-Smith (2006) argues that all "political economies of power" including organizations are "fundamentally relational." That is, power results from relative positions in "[a]n objectified hierarchical order where the distribution of resources and opportunities favors those at the top" (ibid.: 66). As the totality of actors, objects, interests, and institutions are "conditionally constituted," once these relations have been stabilized into predictable and governable relations, they tend to structure "their own and others' futures" (ibid.: 68). In other words, if there is any novelty produced in such durable systems of power, it "[s]prings up from the crevices," Owen-Smith (ibid.: 67) proposes.

Seemingly paradoxical, in this politicized view of institutions, there are thus many opportunities for enterprising behavior and agency at large, activities that aim to either change these instituted relations per se or to identify and exploit these "crevices" in the "durable systems of power." Schmidt et al. (2012: 76) here speak of "Big Politics" (capitalized) as "[a] set of attempts that seek to formally codify and institutionalise *political* decisions, values and actions within collective actors." Big Politics is the political work and processes commonly belonging to the domain of professional jurisdiction of political scientists, the study and analysis of "obdurate networks of ideologies, elections, parliaments, parties, [and] lobby groups – think tanks, trade unions, mayors, and campaigns" (ibid.). In contrast, Schmidt et al. (ibid.) define "micropolitics" as "[a] set of interrelated attempts to open up politics to new actors, to find a space for various others to speak and transform a collective." The micropolitics of institutions belong to the domain of scholarly research of organization researchers, and studies of institutions reveal a form of "Brownian motion" – a term from particle physics denoting how "everything is continually being shaken and jiggled around" on the microscale (Jones, 2004: 13) – in institutions, that is, how they continually modify and procreate to accommodate external social changes.

For instance, Yue, Luo, and Ingram's (2013) study of the elitist Manhattan banking industry reveals that to accomplish the desired stability of the finance industry, continuous change is demanded. Change is operationalized here as the continuous management of "mutual dependence between social groups" to maintain institutional stability (ibid.: 38). In Yue, Luo, and Ingram's (2013) view, regulatory agencies are closely bound up with the finance sector – a claim that has been verified by the literature (see e.g., Blinder, 2013; Mandis, 2013; Cohan, 2011) – and therefore the finance industry actors themselves need to be able to secure the long-term stability of the industry by integrating non-elite actors – what Yue, Luo, and Ingram (2013) refer to as "the out-group" – into the otherwise elite communities controlling the industry:

> Cohesive elites may be tempted to maintain a high level of exclusivity and deny the out-groups equal opportunities for participation in an attempt to monopolize institutional benefits. But elites who succumb to this temptation ignore the fact that the stability of competitive environments rests on a delicate distributional balance with the out-group.
>
> (Yue, Luo, and Ingram, 2013: 39)

The authors explain that if elites gain unbalanced monopoly, this in itself causes the rest of the market conditions to deteriorate, making the influence of market-governance institutions difficult and thus escalating the severity of market crises. In other words, for the enterprising and ambitious out-group actor, there are possibilities for making it into the elite community of Manhattan bankers. This work of the *parvenu* is also beneficial for the elite community as it enables "institutional stabilization." As Yue, Luo, and Ingram (2013: 39) conclude, institutional stabilization is not necessarily an "automatic process" but rather rests on "[o]ngoing mobilization both within the institutionally advantaged group and between them and other social groups." Seemingly paradoxical, institutional stability is accomplished exactly through increased socio-economic diversity, enabling incumbent institutions to gradually adapt to external changes and pressures. Institutional change is therefore only in exceptional cases momentary and conspicuous, as in the case of crises and swift economic changes, while in most cases change occurs at the lower level, at times barely noticed by outsiders. Institutional change is therefore always occurring as a political or at least politicized process wherein the interests of various stakeholders are negotiated and mutually adjusted.

Institutional theory and change

Organizational change as an empirical phenomenon has been something like the Achilles' heel of institutional theory and has created natural boundaries for its colonialist expansion to claim to be able to explain virtually any organizational activity or condition. Institutional theory has historically sought to explain stability, inertia, imitation, and isomorphism both within industries and across organizational fields and markets. In the late-modern regime of competitive capitalism, where ceaseless change and competition are praised not only as factual conditions of the economy but also deemed as the only morally justifiable attitude towards work and renewal, institutional theorists have been at pains to adjust their analytical framework to accommodate also change and renewal.

Change is at times reconceptualized within the incumbent theoretical framework, rendering changes as *deinstitutionalization*. "Deinstitutionalization refers to the process whereby previously institutionalized practices are abandoned," Maguire and Hardy (2009: 150) write. Such a novel theoretical gaze not only comes about "because better options present themselves" but because "practices have lost their original meaning," Maguire and Hardy (ibid.) add. For instance, Davis, Diekmann and Tinskley's (1994: 549) seminal study demonstrates how deregulatory finance market reforms in the Reagan era of the 1980s led to the new possibility of hostile takeovers directed at low valued American conglomerates, leading to the deinstitutionalization of the conglomerate company form and the widely preached portfolio-planning procedures serving to mediate economic downturns and other external shocks that might threaten firm's long-term survival. After hostile takeovers were permitted through more lenient finance market control in combination with the inflow of foreign capital into the high-interest rate American economy in the 1980s (a policy implemented to push down inflation), CEOs and directors became acutely aware of the importance of stock market evaluations of their companies, and business school academics and finance industry pundits started to preach the gospel of "core competencies," the new predominant idea of "specialization" in the 1980s. Taken together, these shifting institutional conditions (political, macroeconomic, ideological, and theoretical) served to deinstitutionalize the conglomerate form (Davis, Diekmann and Tinskley, 1994).

Another case of deinstitutionalization is Eyal's (2013) study of how the psychological condition of autism could be treated in clinical practices only after parents of children with autism, behavioral psychologists, occupational therapists, and other relevant groups could assemble an "alternative network of expertise" that ceased to regard autism as a form of mental illness or retardation but understood autism as a specific condition demanding its own etiology and treatment. In creating these networks of expertise, essentially breaking down the distinction between lay and expert knowledge (ibid.: 867) that child psychologists dominating the field prior to this activism were eager to maintain, autism could be widely recognized and fruitful therapies could be developed. More specifically, the child psychiatrist Leo Kanner who coined the term *autism* in the 1940s played a central role in securing this cooperation with the clients. However, once this institutional shift was in place and autism became embedded in professional practices and beliefs, it became a widespread diagnosis, testifying to the success of the institutional work conducted; by the mid-1960s, Kanner was arguing that autism was being "overdiagnosed" (ibid.: 882).

Both the studies of Davis, Diekmann and Tinskley (1994) and Eyal (2013), despite idiosyncrasies and differences in their cases, emphasize the role of professionals in orchestrating change and processes of deinstitutionalization.

Scott (2008: 223) suggests that professionals, "more so than any other social category," serve the role as "institutional agents," as "definers, interpreters, and appliers of institutional elements." Studies of the historical development of professionals as favored experts or, with a more recent term, knowledge-workers, demonstrates how these groups are capable of claiming jurisdictional authority on the basis of their affiliations with and connections to institutions including guilds, universities, and interests organizations (Larson, 1977; Brint, 1994). Such studies support Scott's (2008) view of professionals as being closely bound up with institutions that legitimize their claims to jurisdictional discretion. In the case where different professional communities or groups are affiliated with the same institutions or are collaborating closely (physicians and nurses being a textbook case), the day-to-day work of professionals are characterized by continuous jurisdictional struggles: "[T]he workplace is a consequential setting for jurisdictional struggles. In hospitals, workplaces with frequent cross-professional interaction, the informal practices and rhetorical strategies of professionals have been shown to blur and alter task boundaries," Bechky (2003: 723) writes. Despite such internal workplace struggles and controversies, professionals remain public spokespersons for the field or industry they represent and spend their careers and working lives serving, and consequently, professionals in many cases act as changers of institutions. Under all conditions, influential professional groups serve as the gatekeepers of institutional fields (Pettigrew, 1973; Corra and Willer, 2002).

For Suddaby and Viale (2011: 426), it is analytically complicated to isolate professionalization projects and processes of institutionalization (i.e., organizational change) as they "occur simultaneously." That is, professional projects are essentially "vehicles of institutionalization and field-level change." As professional groups create, maintain and extend their jurisdictional boundaries, they also, "perhaps unwittingly but often with intent," engage in "processes of institutional work" (ibid.). Professionals extending or securing their jurisdictional discretion thus unfolds as a process of institutionalization. These activities in turn "[r]everberates through the social and organizational fields within which they are situated," Suddaby and Viale (ibid.: 431) argue. This is an analytical model that inscribes a significant amount of agency into professional communities.

In some cases, such a view of professionals as commanding the resources and holding the authority to execute this role as effective institutional actors may be justified, but there are also many studies of how professional communities see their jurisdictional claims being compromised or diminished as new forms of governance are established (e.g., Lorenz, 2012; Currie et al., 2012; Champy, 2006; Kitchener, 2002), e.g., the increasingly popular managerial procedure of auditing (Pentland, 2000; Power, 2003, 1997). In other words, agency on the part of the professional group is more of an empirical question than a theoretical assumption to be made regarding factual conditions in professional fields. Regardless of such concerns, Suddaby and Viale (2011: 437) invite "management scholars" to study professions in greater detail, a domain of research in sociology with long-standing pedigree (Carr-Saunders and Wilson, 1933; Johnson, 1972). In the following, the concept of agency will be further examined and more closely related to the more recent discussions in institutional theory making change and renewal not exceptional events but ongoing and ceaseless processes in organizations.

The concept of agency

One of the standing epistemological issues in the social science literature is the so-called actor–structure problem, that is, how do agency and individual action relate to social structures and communal beliefs and norms. As Sewell (1992: 2) argues, structure tends to be introduced in social scientific discourse as being "impervious to human agency" – to "exist apart from" but nevertheless determining everyday practices of social actors. This is the first theoretical problem, that of how the universal and the particular, the collective and the individual, the whole and the parts, are interrelated and mutually constituted. Second, there is the corollary problem of social change, i.e., how structure and agencies are modified and adapted to new conditions. Many social theorists including Pierre Bourdieu (1977), speaking of the habitus as the agent's internalization of social structures into the habitual schemes directing everyday activities, and Anthony Giddens (1984), who speaks of the recursive and mutually constitutive relationship between structure and agency, have tried to theoretically reconcile structure and agency. In Sewell's (1992: 13) view, structure is composed of the *virtual* element of what he calls *schemas* and the *actual* element of *resources*:

> Structures are at risk, at least to some extent, in all the social encounters they shape – because structures are multiple and intersecting, because schemas are transposable, and because resources are polysemic and accumulate unpredictably. Placing the relationship between resources and cultural schemas at the center of a concept of structure makes it possible to show how social change, no less than social stasis, can be regenerated by the enactment of structures in social life.
>
> (Sewell, 1992: 19)

This is no easily understood passage of social science writing, and perhaps the work of Feldman and Pentland (2003, 2005) on organizational routines – recurrent, standard operation procedures constituting organizations – may shed some light on the relation between virtual and abstract schemas and actual and concrete resources. In Feldman and Pentland's (2003, 2005) view, organizational routines consist of two related parts: first, one "ostensive aspect, the ideal or schematic form of a routine" (Feldman and Pentland, 2005: 96), an abstract and structural part that prescribe practically and normatively how a certain routine should be carried out. The second part is a "performative aspect, specific actions by specific people in specific places and times" (Feldman and Pentland, 2005: 96), i.e., the actual performance of the routine. These two parts, the abstract, virtual, and ostensive scheme of the structure, and the concrete, actual, and performative scheme of the practice are both constitutive elements of the routine. At the same time, Feldman and Pentland (2003: 95) argue, "[n]either parties sufficient to explain (or even describe) the properties of the phenomenon we refer to as 'organizational routines.'" The very concept of organizational routine is thus including these two schemes.

In this model, agency is the performative actualization of virtual communal structures, the practical work accomplished on the basis of abstract principles, norms, and beliefs. Agency is the moment when slumbering social structures come to life, become engaged, and lend themselves to effective action. Sewell states (1992):

> [A]gency arises from the actor's control of resources, which means the capacity to reinterpret or mobilize an array of resources in terms of schemas other than those that constituted the array. Agency is implied by the existence of structure.
>
> (Sewell, 1992: 20)

However, Sewell clarifies that agency only involves some degree of control over the social relations that one is enmeshed in, and that this is dependent on structures and resources: "[A]gents are empowered to act with and against others by structures: they have knowledge of the schemas that inform social life and have access to some measures of human and nonhuman resources. Agency arises from the actor's knowledge of schemas, which means the ability to apply them to new contexts" (Sewell, 1992: 20).

Emirbayer (1998: 970) defines agency as "[t]he temporally constructed engagement by actors of different structural environments – the temporal-rational context of action – which, through the interplay of habit, imagination, and judgment, both reproduces and transforms those structures in interactive response to the problems posed by changing historical situations." This definition does not to the same extent address the concept of structure as Sewell's (1992) does – structures merely seem to be in place and thus need to be recognized and handled – but it is a definition general and inclusive enough to discuss what agency means within an institutional theory framework.

In the social science literature, the concept of agency is widely embraced, becomes more differentiated, and a growing number of non-human entities are consequently inscribed with agency. Social scientists speak of e.g., economic agency (Ross, 1973), socio-technical agency (Preda, 2006), perceptual agency (Monson, 2008), textual agency (Cooren, 2004), and agencies among non-humans (in the actor-network theory framework) including the agency of microbes (Latour, 1988) or scallops (Callon, 1981). In some cases, the concept of agency and its colonization of various domains is disputed (Sayes, 2014; Emirbayer and Mische, 1998), but agency, by and large, seems to be more popular than structuralist theories – not least indicated by the popularity of theories of practice (see e.g., Nicolini, 2013; Bjørkeng, Clegg, and Pistis, 2009; Caroll, Levy, and Richmond, 2008; Carter, Clegg, and Kornberger, 2008) and the concept of sociomaterial practices (Orlikowski, 2007; Styhre et al., 2012). Some commentators argue that this shift towards agency in social science theory has been driven too far in the contemporary cultural climate, emphasizing individualism and the liberal citizen's rights as an autonomous legal subject. Meyer and Jepperson (2000: 100) claim, for instance, that "modern actors" are seen as "autochthonous and natural entities, no longer really embedded in culture."

In institutional theory, historically more concerned with structures and stability than with agency and change, the concept of agency has been rediscovered relatively recently. "As long as institutional theorists mainly concentrated on explaining organizational conformity, the issue of agency was not a central one," Battilana and D'Aunno (2009: 36–37) write. Now, they continue, when institutional theorists have begun to "tackle the issue of change, the question of organizational and human agency has become central." It is important to notice that the institutional theory view of agency is different from the rational actor model – *homo economicus* of neoclassical economic theory (Milonakis and Fine, 2009) – inasmuch as agency is not assumed to be executed in isolation from the wider institutional context. In Battilana and D'Aunno's (2009: 34) view, neoclassical economic theory enacts what Townley (2008: 25) describes as "an extreme view of human agency," treating the human agent as a subject "engaged in the narrow utilitarian pursuit of self-interest," and being stripped of "antecedent associations, history, and attachments." Yet, Townley (2008: 25) continues, this agent is understood as being "sovereign over his or her own choices," in turn based on preferences that "arise mysteriously" (see also Tversky and Kahneman, 1981). In the following, the institutional theory view of agency will be discussed in more detail.

Institutional work and the concept of agency

In organization studies, the literature on institutions are commonly divided into three bodies: (1) classic institutional theory developed primarily in sociology in the interwar and post-World War II period (see e.g., Stinchcombe, 1997; Selznick, 1996); (2) neoinstitutional theory developed from the mid-1970s, increasingly emphasizing "soft issues" such as culture, communication, and symbolism as institutional resources in organizations (e.g., Meyer and Rowan, 1977; DiMaggio and Powell, 1983); and (3) the more recent engagement in institutional theory with agency and practices, stressing that institutions not only enable forms of isomorphism and convergence towards standardized organizational forms but can also engender novelty and change, including innovations and new institutional arrangements. Parsons (1951: 39) defined an *institution* in somewhat circulatory terms as "a complex of institutionalized roles integrated which is of strategic structural significance in the social system in question." In the more recent institutional literature, where agency – as opposed to what Parsons (1951) speaks of as "the social system" – is put forth as a principal theoretical construct to be effectively integrated into a dynamic institutional theory framework, concepts such as *institutional logic* (Thornton and Ocasio, 2008; Friedlander and Alford,

1991), *institutional entrepreneurship* (Battilana, 2006; DiMaggio, 1987), and *institutional work* (Lawrence, Suddaby and Leca, 2009, 2011) have been proposed as viable analytical concepts. These three theoretical concepts will be reviewed in the following paragraphs.

The literature on institutional logic, a term originally introduced by Friedlander and Alford (1991: 248) to denote "a set of material practices and symbolic constructions," is today quite extensive. There are many definitions of the term, arguably stretching from more structurally oriented definitions to definitions that recognize agency. "*Institutional logics* are the socially constructed organizing principles for institutionalized practices in social systems," Nigam and Ocscio (2010: 823) write, representing the former view. Meyer and Hammerschmied (2006) define the term accordingly, speaking quite abstractly about "organizing principles" that guide practices:

> [I]nstitutional logics are the belief systems at play in a social field. They prescribe the organizing principles to guide forms and practice, focus attention, give meaning to activities, and specify what goals and values are to be pursued. They indicate the appropriateness of means, thereby legitimating activities.
>
> (Meyer and Hammerschmied, 2006: 1002)

Third, Thornton (2002: 82) brings institutional logics closer to actual practices when she says that they define "the norms, values, and beliefs that structure the cognition of actors in organizations and provide a collective understanding of how strategic interests and decisions are formulated." This view is quite close to that of Douglas's (1986), assuming that institutions structure and determine the cognition of actors. In the seamless transition from structure to agency, Reay and Hinings (2009: 629) render institutional logics as "the basis of taken-for-granted rules guiding behavior of first-level actors." An institutional logic is "a set of belief systems and associated practices" – the virtual and actual element of Sewell's structure/agency aggregate – that "define the content and meaning of institutions" (ibid.: 631). The term *meaning* is here closely associated with agency as structure has no meaning proper beyond their influence on human action, as in the case of William James's (1975: 123) example of the monetary bank note system, having no foundational meaning beyond its practical function and utility. Dunn and Jones (2010: 114) here speak of institutional logics as the "cultural beliefs and rules that shape the cognition and behaviour of actors."

Thus, while the term institutional logic is structural in its orientation, the logic strongly influences not only the practices of agents but also their ways of thinking, how they perceive the world, and how they construct meaningful identities for themselves (Lok, 2010). Still, organization change comes about when there are shifts in institutional logics that in turn put pressure on actors to modify their practices, cognitive systems, identities, and so forth, to adapt to new conditions. This is a fairly conventional institutional theory view, predicting a capacity of organizations to effectively respond to external changes, in this case writ small on the level of the individual. Organizations adapt to changes and establish new institutional logics that in turn trickle down to the level of the individual.

In the case of *institutional entrepreneurship*, a term first introduced by Princeton sociologist Paul DiMaggio (1987) in his study of culture institutions, things are different as the agent is here portrayed as an enterprising and entrepreneurial figure, not patient enough to await e.g., a shift in institutional logics but rather him or herself being the primus motor of such changes. Conceptually speaking, "institutional entrepreneurship" is an oxymoron as agency is placed in the first room, while the institutional setting is prioritized in the analysis: "Institutional entrepreneurs are actors who have an interest in particular institutional arrangements and who mobilize resources to create new institutions or transform the existing ones," Battilana (2006: 654) explains. Stark also (2009) criticizes institutional theorists for their eagerness to apprehend organization change in society and an economic regime increasingly favoring novelty and change over stability and predictability. In Stark's view (2009: 184), institutional theorists assume that the actors' cognition structure practices and therefore any social action is reduced to what is "taken-for-granted" or an "unreflective activity." Instead, Stark (2009) proposes an entrepreneurship theory model wherein actors instead are assumed to actively reflect upon their practices and conceive of new ways of doing business.

That is, despite the willingness to recognize agency in institutional theory, the theory still remains stuck within a structuralist model of change inasmuch as individual cognition is understood as what changes slowly and only occasionally. In other words, rather than recognizing the foresight and inventiveness of e.g., the entrepreneurs, haphazard events (often playing a key role in producing e.g., technological inventions and scientific findings), institutional theorists overrate the importance of collective and communal shared beliefs and norms as the impetus for change and creation. That is, despite the best intentions, institutional theory slips back to structural explanations – now in the form of norms, beliefs, and shared cognition – of social change.

These concerns and the criticism of putting a rational choice theory of agency in the Trojan horse of institutional entrepreneurship is one of the principal motivators for the concept of *institutional work* being popularized quite recently. Carefully avoiding the rational choice model of agency widely endorsed in neoclassical economic theory (Lounsbury, 2008), while not erasing the human agent entirely, Lawrence, Leca, and Zilber (2013: 1024) suggest that the institutional work literature depicts institutional actors as "[r]eflexive, goal-oriented and capable." In addition, "[i]t focuses on actors' actions as the centre of institutional dynamics, and it strives to capture structure, agency, and their interrelations" (Lawrence, Leca, and Zilber, 2013). As a consequence, institutional work is defined as "purposive action aimed at affecting institutions" (Lawrence, Leca, and Zilber, 2013: 1029). The term *purposive action* here needs to be understood in the light of previous critique of the belief in such unrestrained forms of agency (see e.g., Merton, 1936), and Lawrence, Leca, and Zilber (2013: 1029) therefore assure that the widespread view of actors in institutional theory as being experts capable of "[s]killfully manipulating their institutional environments" tend to underestimate the cognitive and emotional efforts demanded to accomplish institutional change.

Therefore, institutional work is not based on a romantic view of individual actors as singlehandedly being able to overcome all kinds of resistance and inertia; institutional work is better seen as a form of "muddling through" (Lindblom, 1959) or a "mangle of practice" (Pickering, 1993) – a form of goal-oriented action beset by many unpredictable events and unanticipated outcomes (Merton, 1936). In this view, institutions are indeed changed, but the consequences of purposive action need to be understood not so much as enterprising activities as the joint work to mutually adjust a variety of institutional and individual interests. That is, institutional work is an analytical concept that enacts a socially embedded view of agency (Granovetter, 1985):

> The concept of institutional work highlights the intentional actions taken in relations to institutions, some highly visible and dramatic, as often illustrated in research on institutional entrepreneurship, but much of it nearly invisible and often mundane, as in the day-to-day adjustments, adaptations, and compromises of actors attempting to maintain institutional arrangements. Thus, a significant part of the promise of institutional work as a research area is to establish a broader vision of agency in relationship to institutions, one that avoids depicting actors either as 'cultural dopes' trapped by institutional arrangements, or as hypermuscular institutional entrepreneurs.
>
> (Lawrence, Suddaby and Leca, 2009: 1)

In the field of reproductive medicine and ART, such a view of institutionally embedded agency is helpful in understanding how scientific, economic, financial, and ethical concerns and interests can be negotiated, aligned, and mutually adjusted to develop clinical practices and accompanying policies and regulatory frameworks that effectively balances opportunities, risk, and concerns and that can be accepted and tolerated by a majority of the stakeholders. As the empirical material reported in Part II of this volume will demonstrate, in the case of e.g., social freezing, very much a clinical service being a direct consequence of changing social behavior, and new career patterns and work life opportunities for women, there are a variety of issues and concerns regarding the development of additional commercial reproductive services. That is, institutional work is never really finally accomplished as soon as a new position has been entrenched, but previous beliefs and objections – e.g., the idea of naturalness of human reproduction – tend to be rearticulated in new terms as soon as new issues are addressed and new opportunities are presented.

The three forms of institutional work

Lawrence, Suddaby and Leca (2009: 8–9) define three forms of institutional work: (1) "creating institutions"; (2) "maintaining institutions"; and (3) "disrupting institutions." In the analysis of ART and reproductive medicine, this elementary triptych will be used to shed light on how a field of expertise is related to and accommodates new innovations, practices, technologies, and concepts that in turn serve to renew and maintain the interest among professional groups, policy-makers and other relevant social groups. This joint work to create new opportunities, in many cases on the basis of technoscientific and biomedical expertise, will be referred to as institutional work that creates new institutions. Second, any institutional or professional field needs routines and standard operation procedures to be able to subsist over time. There is a need for clinical routines structured into protocols, standards for negotiating and bargaining formal contracts, and more practical standards for e.g., accounting and economic control procedures. In maturing industries much of this institutional maintenance work occurs outside of the public gaze, not because this work is not interesting but because it is part of the run-of-the-mill activities that barely interests the wider public. As will be demonstrated in Chapter 7, much of the institutional maintenance work today takes place in private firms and in private clinics that serve the Swedish public health care sector. As a consequence, relations between privately owned corporations and public sector organizations, ultimately determined by political interests, needs to be harmonious and characterized by a great deal of mutual understanding and adjustment to align various interest and institutional differences. Third and finally, there is a form of institutional work that actively seeks to question or even overturn existing institutional norms, beliefs, or practices. While the creation of institutions to a large extent is the privilege of centrally located professional groups such as, in this case, researchers in reproductive medicine or gynecologists and obstetricians with clinical know-how, the disruption of institutions is more frequently caused by outsiders. Outsiders is here a quite heterogeneous group including entrepreneurs seeking to exploit unchartered territories in a market or customer interest groups that call for a change to meet some emerging and to date overlooked social demand. The work to disrupt institutions is therefore what basically emerges in the organization's environment and therefore is an exogenous factor that needs to be adapted to.

The three forms of institutional work are not of necessity mutually excluding and the line of demarcation of the three categories is porous and fluid, making it difficult to maintain a clear-cut and unproblematic definition of the three forms of institutional work. Seen in this way, the three-pronged institutional work model is not based on the idea of theoretical purity but is better understood as what can help the analyst make sense of and structure messy and complex data. This is precisely how the concepts of Lawrence, Suddaby and Leca (2009) have been put to work in this study, to structure the analysis of a field that is today maturing but that still is in a perpetual process of change as there are new technologies and techniques developed, new social issues to consider, and new interest groups raising their voices. ART and reproductive medicine is still in a stage of developing and changing, yet it is firmly rooted in the legal and regulatory framework that structure the activities and the clinical practices in day-to-day work. This ongoing balancing of renewal and stability, innovation and control, constant modification to adapt to new social needs and regulatory transparency demands makes the concept of institutional work a helpful analytical model.

3   The science of reproductive medicine and the market for assisted reproductive technologies

Introduction

In the discourse about human reproduction over the last half century, the increasing rate of out of wedlock births has been a concern for those taking on the role of defending the traditional family structure. In the U.S., between 1960 and 1979 there was more than a twofold increase in divorce rates, and the fertility rates of women has fallen from its peak in the mid-1950s (Markens, 2007: 10). By 1990, over 25 percent of births were to unmarried women, compared to only 5 percent in 1960 and today, Goodwin (2010: 5) writes, "Nearly 40 percent of births in the United States are to unwed mothers," accounting for a 25 percent rise in just five years. Moreover, between the 1960s and 1992, the proportion of children living in single-mother families "almost tripled (from 8 percent to 23 percent)" (Markens, 2007: 10). For guardians of the historically predominant family structure, the nuclear heterosexual family including one or more kids, such statistics are daunting as it indicates that "the nuclear family" is in crisis.

In addition to the concerns that fewer children grow up in these "traditional family structures," other commentators have added that the postponement of parenting and mothering in particular to the 30s and beyond the age of 35 is partially explained on the basis of the "tertiary-education-and-career" work life choices that especially middle class women make. These women and their spouses, male as well as female, also encounter a working life situation that is unwelcoming for aspiring parents, Briggs notices:

> [Reproductive technology] is addressing structural infertility and a considerable increase in difficulty in getting pregnant caused by the fact that, on the whole, many middle class women are being forced by family-unfriendly workplaces and educational institutions to delay childbearing until their thirties and beyond (and not just in the United States).
>
> (Briggs, 2010: 373)

As Hochschild (1997) has persuasively argued, the last decades' increased competition in society and not least in the deregulated competitive capitalist economic system has abandoned the interwar and post-World War II period ideal of the "family man" (as there were few career women prior to the 1960s, the "family woman" never got stuck as a gendered stereotype in American popular culture). The family man has moved from being praised as an admirable social position, testifying to maturity and the ability to carry responsibilities, to a position where the term has "taken on negative overtones, designating a worker who isn't a serious player" (Hochschild, 1997: 113). If nothing else, the extensive literature on how to balance work life and family life (e.g., Watts, 2009; Perlow, 1998) is indicative of this shift. In order to effectively balance an American work credo (see Schor, 1993) with a reasonably functional family life, there is today a large and expanding market for professional household services taking care of issues such as birthday parties for the children or the "management" of social relations with friends and family, previously being included in the private life sphere (Hochschild, 2012). The more widespread use of such services make family life resemble companies, where "make or buy" decisions and decisions on what activities to "outsource" become actual choices to make. Following this line of argument, indicative of isomorphisms across the work life/family divide, Hochschild (1997: 219) speaks of "Taylorized children" in the case of children growing up in families where "time famine" (Perlow, 1999) is endemic and mediated by the recourse to various market-based services. ART is described as one of these services that many families are more or less forced to make use of: "It's not a particularly effective, often hugely expensive Band-Aid on a considerable loss of reproductive choice in the last forty years" (Briggs, 2010: 373).

In these accounts, there is both evidence of new preferences, opportunities, and beliefs regarding desirable family formations and an increasingly more demanding work life that claim its casualties in terms of couples and single women becoming aware that they are not as fertile as they expected, thus making assisted reproduction therapies and technologies an option to fulfill their dream of becoming parents. Today, it is estimated that 10 percent of the American population suffer from infertility problems (Almeling, 2007), and there is no reason to believe the figure should be lower in any comparative country. In a global perspective, infertility affects approximately 80 million women and men worldwide (Inhorn and Birenbaum-Carmeli, 2008: 179), but many of these would never be able to afford costly IVF therapies. Social and cultural changes have liberated women and offer them a wider set of life chances and opportunities. One consequence is that women therefore need to make hard decisions of whether to postpone parenting during their early careers. Fortunately, these social changes and their tendency to increase infertility problems have been counteracted by the advancement of technoscientific know-how and practices, available to some.

This chapter will review the literature on assisted reproductive technologies and stresses how the widespread use and recognition of e.g., ART is a quite recent phenomenon. In addition, the development of reproductive medicine and the various clinical practices, today helping thousands of couples and single women overcome their "natural" infertility, has by no means been straightforward or devoid of criticism, politics, and ethical concerns. Instead, assisted reproductive technologies is a human accomplishment in the purest meaning of the term, representing both the physiological discovery of the elementary processes of human reproduction on the molecular and cellular levels and the social and cultural shift towards a more forgiving and liberal view of sexuality, families and parenting. In addition, the development of assisted reproductive technologies is based on institutional, organizational, and managerial developments, making access to the therapies widespread and available at a relatively low cost in many developed countries providing public health care services.

The concept of biomedicalization

Modern medicine and the branch of reproductive medicine is the outcome from the convergence of a variety of disciplinary development and changes for more than two centuries beginning around the year 1800. Chemistry offers an analytical framework for the molecular structure of the genome of humans and other biological organisms, and biology and medicine provide integrative theories about the human biological organism and its reproductive capacities. In order to fully capture the full complexity of modern biomedical technosciences and its clinical application, the term *biomedicine* is helpful as it includes laboratory research work, clinical practices, and the regulatory system that frames these activities. Mamo (2007: 369) defines biomedicine loosely as "a set of diverse institutions, discourses, and practices, [that] shapes the meaning and experiences of technological use." The accompanying term *biomedicalization*, developed by Adele Clarke, Laura Mamo and their colleagues, in turn "[e]ncompasses the cumulative impact and cultural pervasiveness of technoscience, as well as a focus on risk and surveillance, a rise in lifestyle and customized medicines, and other social processes that take place as medicine travels in new ways and into new places" (ibid.: 370). Biomedicalization is thus both a set of practices, methods, and skills, but also a regime of governance in the era of advanced biopolitics.

Biomedicalization as a form of governance therefore not only examines and treats the body proper in the unfortunate case of illness or injury but actively engages in creating what Berg and Bowker (1997: 514) speak of as "the medical body" and contributes to what Sharp (2011: 7) speaks of as "body tinkering," the systematic work to not only explore but also to enhance and modify the human body. In many cases, this work is conducted with the best of intentions to help humans e.g., defeat cancer, cardiac arrests, or sub-fertility, but there is also a significant literature that speaks of medicalization and biomedicalization as the unwarranted expansion of medical therapies and consumption of drugs on the basis of commercial interests rather than medical needs and adequate health care concerns and recommendations (Dumit, 2012; Abraham, 2010; Shostak and Conrad, 2008; Blech, 2006). In addition, in the case of reproductive medicine and assisted reproduction technologies, scholars and feminist activists have been critical of how the female reproductive capacities to some extent have been "expropriated" by commercial interests, represented by privately owned IVF clinics and international egg agencies, and surrogacy clinics. The concepts of biomedicine and biomedicalization thus effectively accommodates both the promises and the concerns of late-modern biomedical technoscience, and do not sweep issues of power, politics, and authority under the carpet.

The troubled feminist reception of assisted reproduction therapies also need to be understood within a tradition of civil rights activism where, as Ertman (2010: 32) remarked, women's entrenched status as "full citizens and legal subjects" is of quite recent date. One may here add that in the field of ART, this is a very accurate reminder. Women's rights as full citizens have been entrenched relatively recently, and women have historically also been closely associated – primarily by male professionals and authorities – with various forms of embodied and biological processes, including the menstruation cycle and their reproductive capacities, and consequently the treatment of women as "baby-factories," recalls an uncanny past that feminist scholars and activists need to be conscious about, yet want to treat as outmoded ways of thinking. Under all conditions, regardless of the clinical benefits of assisted reproduction technologies, the feminist-informed literature on this matter oscillates between an affirmative recognition of reproductive medicine as a liberating project (Murphy, 2012) and more skeptical accounts (Twine, 2011).

Reproductive medicine as practice and science

In the analysis of how reproductive medicine has been developed, it is helpful to distinguish between on the one hand the private everyday concern to monitor and regulate individual fertility, especially in societies taking a grim and moralist view of undisciplined sexual liberties, not least for unmarried women, and the scholarly and academic development of a discipline of sexual reproduction. To start with, it will make no fuss to say that human reproduction and human sexuality as biological drives and capacities have been very influential in all human societies (Ginsburg and Rapp, 1991). While anthropological studies reveal a quite playful and relaxed view of sexuality and reproduction, in e.g., Melanie Klein's study of sexual practices in Micronesia, in the Christian West, at least after the medieval period that was characterized by relatively lower degrees of social control (Elias, 1978), sexuality and reproduction has been a key occupation for the clergy, various authorities, and moralists. Especially in the bourgeoisie society emerging after the "two revolutions of modernity," the political revolution in France – commonly treated by historians as the starting point for the modern period (Wallerstein, 2011) – and the Industrial Revolution, being the ultimate evidence of the bourgeoisie's triumph over outmoded Aristocratic ways of life, embedded in conspicuous consumption and leisure activities rather than hard and venturesome work, sexuality became something like an obsession.

As Foucault examines in his three-volume work on the history of sexuality (Foucault, 1978, 1980, 2000), there has been no period more preoccupied with sexuality than the modern period. Strong sentiments and in many cases repressive and unforgiving morals, making primarily women victims of their own biologically endowed drives and instincts, was fertile ground for double standards and an operative distinction between official morals and private practices and liberties. For instance, the Christian taboo against replicating Onan's sin to waste semen – an idea of Greek origin, Foucault (1978) shows – made masturbation shameful and was claimed to damage the male adolescent's physical features. At the same time, such taboos did not prevent bourgeoisie fathers from giving their sons money to spend in brothels to "release their sexual tensions." That is, masturbating was sinful but to seek the assistance of prostitutes, unfortunate women enduring harrowing lives and that frequently served to spread diseases such as syphilis, was not frowned upon, at least not outside of the more official and formal circles (Gay, 2001).

As detailed by Gay (2001), in the Victorian bourgeoisie culture, reproduction was a sacred domain and procreation was sanctioned by the bible, yet human sexuality was thoroughly regulated and controlled. Population alarmists in e.g., Germany and the United States were concerned about falling birth rates and the American Theodore Roosevelt used the term "race suicide" when addressing the issue (ibid.: 53). As a consequence, any attempt to control birth and to interfere with possible pregnancy was treated as "unnatural" (ibid.: 52). At the same time, sexual drives and needs and the coitus that precede the pregnancy were not acclaimed as equally "natural" and worthy of encouragement, creating a curious and confusing blend of encouragement, mystification, and moralism surrounding human reproduction. As contraception was banned in e.g., the U.S., the Victorian era was dominated by *coitus interruptus* or what was widely addressed as "withdrawal" to prevent undesired pregnancies, a method that especially many unwed younger women learned the hard way to be unreliable (ibid.: 54). There were a variety of contraceptives including "vaginal jellies, douches, or pessaries" (ibid.: 55) offered in the period but such resources were expensive and complicated to acquire. Fortunately, the wonders of science and inventiveness gave a helping hand, and Charles Goodyear's invention of the vulcanization of rubber in 1839 led to a drop in prices of condoms by the 1860s (ibid.: 55). In the U.S., contraceptives became illegal by 1879, leading to this "flourishing industry" going underground. As late as 1938, when contraceptives were still illegal, "products with virtually no name" generated annual revenues of "roughly 250 million dollars" in the U.S. (Spar, 2010: 182–183).

Moralist sentiments regarding human sexuality and its consequences seemed to counteract individual desires and sexual practices poorly. In the Victorian era, there was thus a harsh struggle between the moral authorities that regarded birth as not only natural but also a Christian duty – "marry and multiply" was the dictum – and everyday people trying to navigate in this most difficult terrain, were beset by both biological and emotional needs and a series of taboos, sins, and dangers. Needless to say, this was unchartered territory for especially younger women whose sexuality could only be legitimately recognized within the safe haven of marriage. It is perhaps no wonder that the development of the contraceptive pill was financially supported by feminist activist groups, eager to create possibilities for women to individually control and monitor their reproductive capacities (Watkins, 2001).

Regardless of these concerns regarding human reproduction, there was relatively little know-how about its biology. In 1892, a zoologist at the University of Lyon, an authority of the day, wrote that, "Our knowledge of the nature of the intimate phenomenon of fecundation is of quite recent origin" (cited in Gay, 2001: 57). In addition, issues of sexuality were not included in the health care apparatus until relatively late. In 1910, Margaret Sanger coined the term "birth control," and in the 1970s, "reproductive health" was more widely used, being "crystallized" into a governance term by the early 1990s (Murphy, 2013: 8). Clarke's (1990) study of the historical development of reproductive medicine reveals how a variety of professional fields and interests converged, including development in veterinary medicine, endocrinology, cellular medicine, and gynecology and obstetrics, led to the systematic study of human reproduction. In many cases the explicit intentions were to monitor and control reproductive capacities – a goal justified by the recent "population explosion" discourse of the post-World War II period (see also Shaw, 2012).

In veterinary medicine and in the breeding of cattle, there was at an early stage an understanding of the economic value of knowing how to optimize the quality of the stock, and some of its know-how regarding inheritance was translated into reproductive medicine. "Reproductive sciences were embedded within and dependent upon industrialization processes that enhanced control over nature and social life," Clarke (1990: 34) writes. In the field of embryology, derived from veterinary medicine and its interest in heredity factors, Walter Heape conducted embryo transfer experiments in the U.K. between 1890 and 1899, and by the first decades of the new century, there was an important shift in embryology research from "mere observation" via dissection or classification to a more "direct interference" with the internal mechanisms of the embryo (Franklin, 2014: 114). These changes were also accompanied by new theoretical developments such as the so-called *Entwicklungsmechanik*, the "development mechanics" of embryos, advanced by the German and Swiss embryologists Wilhelm Roux and Wilhelm His, seeking to unravel the biological differentiation of the embryo during its growth. This shift in theory and methodology were summarized in the textbook *Experimental Embryology* published by J.W. Jenkinson in 1909.

In the 1930s, Gregory Pincus tried to create IVF practices in animals at Cambridge University, dubbed "the Pincogenesis," leading to a number of "stem technologies" being fused in this attempt (Franklin, 2014: 132). In Pincus's work, it became increasingly complicated to separate the components: "[T]he differences between what is biological, what is a biological mechanism, what is an experimental system, and what is an experimental tool are deliberately rendered opaque," Franklin (ibid.: 133) writes. The early form of IVF thus took the form of biological engineering where "the biology only works when it is coupled to the right tools" (ibid.: 133). Both Gregory Pincus and his successor Robert Edwards were "iconoclastic, antiestablishment, and controversial biological engineers," sharing the commitment to enable social progress through the control of the early stages of life (ibid.: 135).

In the 1950s and 1960s, Robert G. Edwards worked in a number of different fields including embryology and genetics, and until 1968 his principal research interest was to use *preimplantation genetic diagnosis* to reveal Down, Klinefelter, and Turner syndromes in human embryos (Johnson, 2011). When Edwards wanted to take Pincus's research further – these two pioneers met once at a conference in Venice in May 1966 (Johnson, 2011: 246) – and fertilize human ova in the laboratory and transfer the grown embryo to the womb to enable pregnancies in infertile women, gynecologists that were informed about the project "candidly responded they thought the idea preposterous," Edwards (2001: 1091) writes. Edwards also encountered criticism from ethicists, "forecasting abnormal babies, misleading the infertile and misrepresenting our work as really acquiring human embryos for research" (ibid.: 1092). In addition, which appears as an odd argument today, these critics "announced that IVF did not cure infertility, as women remained infertile after having an IVF baby" (ibid.: 1092).

As Johnson (2011) writes, it is complicated to understand today, more than four decades later, what kind of resistance Edwards and his colleagues encountered in the 1960s but one should keep in mind that infertility was not officially recognized as a disease category by the World Health Organization until as late as 1993 (Mamo, 2007: 30). The British Medical Research Council did not recognize infertility at all among its targeted research areas, and overpopulation and family planning were seen as "dominant concerns" in the period (ibid.: 258). In addition to the neo-Malthusian fear of overpopulation, a fair share of Victorian and Edwardian era misogyny lingered on. As detailed by Pfeffer (1999), by the turn of the twentieth century, clinical gynecology was both surrounded by the anxieties that male sexuality and female sexuality in particular caused in the period, and common sense thinking moralizing e.g., sterility:

> Sterility was considered the price paid by women for slack moral habits. Women who led a worthless life, filled with idleness, sensuality and rich food, were less fertile than hard-working women who are simply fare. Sexualized and sexually active women – epitomized by prostitutes – who took great many hot baths, rose at ten or eleven in the morning, and generally led an 'animal life,' rarely had children.
>
> (Pfeffer, 1999: 33)

As a consequence, in the community of physicians, gynecologists were "seen as parvenus and faced an uphill struggle to wrest control of women's bodies from both physician *accoucheurs* and abdominal surgeons," Pfeffer (1999: 42) writes: "In fact, gynaecology was considered to be one of the most controversial fields in medicine." Based on such historical records, even in the late 1960s, "the infertile were ignored as, at best, a tiny and irrelevant minority and at worst as a positive contribution to population control" (Johnson, 2011: 258). Edwards and his colleagues thus encountered the most insidious form of resistance, that of common sense (see e.g., Koyré, 1968: 12). Edwards refused to accept this value system and his political views – Edwards was born into a working-class Yorkshire family – "demanded that he fought the corner of the infertile: the underdog with no voice" (Johnson, 2011: 258). Edwards also received many encouraging letters from infertile couples, which "spurred him on and provided a major stimulus to his continued work later, despite so much professional and press antagonism" (ibid.).

One of the principal concerns for Edwards was how to secure the access to human ova as scientists were not permitted to retrieve eggs from female patients, but he created alliances with gynecologists that shared his commitment to the research project. Edwards and his collaborators' long and persistent work during close to three decades was in a way accomplished when the first baby fertilized in the laboratory, Louise Brown, was born on July 26, 1978. "It is hard to put into words what the occasion of her [Louise Brown's] birth meant to me, and to our wonderful supportive team. It was purely routine caesarian section, yes, but with a significance outstripping anything we had done before or were likely to achieve later," Edwards (2001: 1093) recalls.

In the course of the development of experimental embryology and biology at large, there was an increased emphasis on the molecular levels of the cell after World War II (Fujimura, 2006; Rheinberger, 2000), representing a "molecular paradigm" (Neumann-Held and Rehmann-Sutter, 2006) enacting the embryo as an informational structure with specific developmental pathways. More recently, the interest has shifted from the human genome per se and genomics methods, to novel biomedical concepts such as proteomics (Myers, 2008), serving to undermine what Neumann-Held (2006) speaks of as DNA's "ontological privilege" in post-World War II biomedicine research and to widen the scope of the analytical gaze. The more strict scholarly interests also blended with more social concerns in the first decades of the twentieth century, and the modern birth control movement in the U.S. and elsewhere started as a "progressive movement to enhance women's control over their reproductive capacities" (Clarke, 1990: 34). The very same expertise that was developed to curb human reproduction to counteract global population growth was used to advance its opposite objective – to overcome human infertility and to give birth to babies on the basis of assisted reproduction.

The research program initiated by Robert Edwards in the U.K. and elsewhere to develop what would be widely known as in vitro fertilization was both regarded with fear and skepticism. Derogatory terms such as "baby-factories" were used to disqualify the research work and Aldous Huxley's term "test-tube babies" introduced in his chilling dystopia *A Brave New World* (1932), where babies are designed and produced on industrial basis to satisfy social demands was dusted off to demonize Edwards and others. Fortunately, the efficacy and safety of the new therapy served to overcome these early fears and quite understandable concerns. As quick as 1986, only five years after the first American IVF "test-tube baby" Elizabeth Jordan Carr was born in December 1981, IVF was "nearly routine" and was no longer "vilified" (Spar, 2010: 184). By 2003, less than two decades later, "there were 437 clinics in the United States, which reported 112,872 cycles and producing, as a result, 48,756 babies" (ibid.). Despite fighting common sense norms about the virtues of "natural births" and not least concerns regarding the physical and psychological features of the babies fertilized in the laboratory, and widespread concern among policy-makers regarding over-populations, the pioneers of assisted reproduction developed and successfully introduced the first clinical method helping sub-fertile couples and women become parents.

As Franklin (2014) emphasizes, the history of reproductive medicine and its clinical branch assisted reproduction is characterized by its hybridity, its ability to align and bring into harmony a variety of professional skills and know-how, social and financial interests, stakeholders and activists groups, and to bridge private and public interests. In short, IVF is constituted as an assemblage and therefore much of the know-how developed can be used in parallel scientific endeavors. In Franklin's phrasing, IVF has evolved from being "an experimental research technique used in embryology" into "a global technological platform" that can be used in a wide variety of applications, from "genetic diagnoses and livestock breeding to cloning and stem cell research" (ibid.: 1–2). In other words, in vitro fertilization is at once "a technique, a model, an imitation of a biological process, synthesis process, a scientific research method, and agricultural tool, and a means of human reproduction – of making life" (ibid.: 3).

At the same time, all these biomedical technoscientific possibilities and applications mingle with social conditions and beliefs including ideas about "naturalized and normalized logic of kinship, parenthood, and reproduction" (Franklin, 2014: 4). As a consequence, assisted reproduction technologies and clinical practices are "a science of the intimate," of perhaps the most private sphere of human life, that of sexuality and reproduction, in many cases surrounded by strong collective moral norms and personal beliefs, at the same time as it provokes worries and anxiety as it actively manipulates human reproductive resources. This makes assisted reproduction technologies a most complex domain of social practice, both from a practical and analytical perspective, as it cuts through conventional boundaries between nature and culture, private and public, common sense thinking and professional expertise, naturalness and artifice.

The clinical perspective: assisted reproduction technologies and the pursuit of human reproduction

Definitions, controversial views, and debates

For many social theorists and scholars informed by feminist theory in particular, Assisted Reproductive Technologies (ARTs) is a complicated matter, dual as they are in terms of their ability to both liberate and exploit human reproductive capacities. Like many other biomedical practices, ART are at their essence representative of the distinction between the two forms of power identified by Spinoza, translated into *pouvoir* and *puissance* by Foucault; *pouvoir* being the progressive power or ability to accomplish things, to create and to become; *puissance* being the regressive or repressive power to dominate and control others. For many theorist commentators, ART is thus Janus-faced inasmuch as it simultaneously enables sub-fertile women and couples to become parents, yet they reduce the female reproductive capacities to a set of interrelated, yet distinctively separable resources and processes. Hammons (2008: 270) thus suggests that ART involves "the commodification of processes of reproduction and motherhood." At the same time, Hammons (ibid.) suggests, in traditional common sense thinking, females tend to not be viewed as "true women," or at least not "adult women" until they become mothers, i.e., implicitly or explicitly "motherhood is seen as intrinsic to adult female identity." As ART have the capacity to separate "the biological from the social," ART have the potential to challenge such images of motherhood by "de-emphasizing genetic ties and elevating the importance of social ones" (ibid.). Also Goslinga-Roy (2000: 113) shares this view of ART: "A common theme in the feminist literature on the reproductive technologies has been that their advent has disarticulated reproduction into its genetic, biological and social aspects."

This view of ART places feminist theory-informed scholars in the position where they on the one hand recognize the discourse on "natural human reproduction" in their critique of ART as being inherently exploitative, while on the other hand embracing the separation between "biological" and "social" motherhood as a source of liberation for women, for generations tied to their physical bodies in their making of social identities. For these scholars, ART is what Plato speaks of as a *pharmakon*, a *potion* in the dialogue *Phaedrus* (Plato, 1995), it is simultaneously a remedy and a poison and therefore one must address ART with great care. At the same time, occasionally feminist theory-informed scholars succumb to common sense thinking when advancing the argument that ART and reproductive medicine more broadly exploits human reproduction in a world characterized by overpopulation and an excess of children on the global scale: "There is something terribly unbalanced about pouring millions of dollars in an effort to enable a small number of privileged women (or the men whose wives they are) to procreate, when there are thousands if not millions of children in need of adoptive or foster homes," Longino (1992: 333) argues. Such arguments have accompanied reproductive medicine and its clinical application since their inception, in many cases in combination with versions of what nature is and how nature is supposedly constituted and reproduced. At the same time, scholarly investigations rarely gain their impetus from common sense thinking but from active explorations and critical self-correction, while it must constantly – for good reasons – respond to common sense objections.

Despite these debates, several different types of clinical practice flourish under the umbrella term ART. Hammons (2008: 270) defines four categories of ARTs: *traditional surrogacy, gestational surrogacy, in vitro fertilization*, and *egg donation*. These new clinical practices either substitute existing practices as in the case of uterus transplant surgery reducing the demand for surrogacy, or complement existing therapies as in the case of PGS and in vitro fertilization. In the following sections, these three ART and their clinical practices will be examined, beginning with the most widespread and least controversial practice of IVF and ending with technoscientific research projects in the field of reproductive medicine that are still at a basic research level but that hold a promise for the future.

The market for gametes: donating eggs and cashing in on sperm samples

As we argued in the Introduction to this book, ART are not always easily embedded in market relations. On the one hand, an "overregulation" may easily marginalize the interest of minority groups and leave the majority's inherited morals and lay theories about reproduction as an all too strong influence on the legislation (Ertman, 2010); on the other hand, a "free-market policy" can easily lead to the exploitation of both donors and would-be parents, and unregulated market transactions may potentially violate norms regarding what human capacities and resources could be subject to market valuation and pricing. In many developed countries, the "market for reproduction" (Spar, 2010: 179) has developed into a combination of public health care services and private enterprise, including both "gift giving" and more straightforward profit motives on the part of the actors. The market for gametes, eggs and sperm, is one area where this hybrid form of planned health care and open market transactions are combined in interesting ways.

Richard Titmuss's (1970) seminal study of blood donation strongly advocated a public sector organization of blood supply, rooted in a *Gemeinschaft* ideology wherein individuals participate in gift giving on the basis of a strong sense of being included in social communities and the obligation to contribute to public well-being. In Titmuss's account, a gift economy-based market for blood and blood plasma would reduce costs and increase the quality of the blood, not least because it would not attract individuals desperate to sell their blood as a source of quick and reliable income, which in turn would increase the demand for quality control and induce additional safety concerns. Needless to say, much neoliberal and pro-business water has flowed under the policy bridges since 1970, and today planned and collectivistic economic activities are perhaps no longer as widely acclaimed and trusted as in 1970, one of the very last years of the post-World War II expansion of the Keynesian welfare state. Despite the comprehensive institutional and policy changes since 1970, many of Titmuss's (1970) arguments are convincing, and there is for instance in many cases an altruistic or social component in all donations at the same time as the financial motives should not be underrated (Almeling, 2011).

In the U.S., the market for gametes include both commercial agencies and banks and agencies being run on the basis of social activist agendas (Mamo, 2007; Simonds, 1996), in many cases founded by feminist groups (Almeling, 2011). The American market for "egg and sperm sales" is largely unregulated and thus offers a "relatively free, open market in which most middle-class people can participate" (Ertman, 2010: 26). Currently, the U.S. market prices the gametes accordingly: Men receive $75 for a sperm donation, and women get paid $4,000 (*New York Times*, May 15, 2007, cited in Ertman [2010: 28]. Cahn [2010: 147] reports the same price for egg but prices sperm at $100), a pricing that represents both the supply and the ordeal demanded from female donors who need to both undergo hormone therapies and the not entirely pleasant procedure where the eggs are retrieved from the ovaries. In Mitchell and Waldby's (2010: 339) vocabulary, female egg donors engage in *intensive clinical labor* while e.g., blood or sperm donors engage with *extensive clinical labor*. In addition, while sperm may not be treated as a renewable biological material, it does not play the same role for male donors as the eggs do for female donors and the regulation of their menopause, i.e., female eggs remain the more limited biological resource. Third and finally, the price paid arguably reflects social and cultural norms regarding gendered views of gametes, where females must guard and protect their reproductive capacities whereas men can at a lower social cost spare their "sex cells."

It is noteworthy that in the market for gametes, there are not only strong ethnic and racial preferences, in many cases quite understandable as it may be preferable for would-be parents to raise children that look similar to themselves, which would also spare them a bit of questioning and answering regarding the biographies of their children. However, these preferences also include much common sense thinking and lay theories about the nature of inheritance. Most life science researchers accept a distinction between what Keller (2010) speaks of as "nature" and "nurture," the influence of both the hereditary material ("nature") and socio-economic and biological environment wherein the child is raised ("nurture"), and few researchers believe that the hereditary material determinate e.g., social skills and competencies as much of these skills can be trained. Recent neurological research also demonstrates a remarkable plasticity of e.g., the human brain, indicating that humans are receptive to learning and motivational factors throughout their lives (Changeux, 2004; Pitts-Taylor, 2010). Still, recipients of human eggs and sperm are prone to inscribe certain desired qualities into these undifferentiated cells, which create good market opportunities for primarily certain female donors to sell their eggs:

> Egg market pricing … is highly differentiated according to the perceived genetic quality and traits of the egg-donor. As the market has become more commercial, the demand for particular genetic preferences has increased. Although the baseline rate for eggs in 1999 was twenty-five hundred to five-thousand dollars, depending on geographic region, donors with traits that are particularly rare or desired commend significantly higher prices. For instance, East Asian and Jewish eggs command a price premium because they are rarer, as do eggs of Ivy League college students, women with high SAT scores, women with athletic ability, and women with extraordinary physical attractiveness.
>
> (Krawiec, 2010: 43)

As Elster (2010: 231) remarks, the selection of gametes thus complies with the same preferences demonstrated when humans select a mate with whom to reproduce, making the gamete selection what is influenced by what is arguably primordial biological instincts rather than a "rational" choice. That is, recipients cannot take into account that these gametes cannot be used to predict whether the future child will become a Nobel Prize Laureate, an athlete sports star, a drug-user, or a just a regular, average Tom, Dick, or Harriet. In some cases, these preferences articulated by the recipients of gametes border to what is mildly amusing as too high expectations are inscribed into these tiny biological entities: "As one US professor confidentially revealed to me, her donors matched very specific preferences not only by race, eye color, and hair color, but also the superfluous, such as vocal accent (the donor was British)" (Goodwin, 2011: 838).

Despite being very human to ask oneself, "Do the sperm speak scouse?," the tendency to project desired qualities onto the gametes may lead to certain donors, primarily women, being undercompensated for their clinical labor. Elster (2010: 234) suggests that there seems to be "some injustice" when an attractive Ivy-league student can earn tens of thousands of dollars donating her eggs to an affluent rich infertile couple, while a single mom on welfare, undergoing the same therapy and procedure, is only eligible to donate for research and thus only reimbursed for actual expenses simply because of her social standing. The proponents of free-market solutions to the exchange of gametes see things differently and on the contrary believe that the Ivy-league student is being discriminated in the regulated market, preventing the more attractive donor capitalizing on her very own achievements and biological qualities. Needless to say, these two opposing views are not easily reconciled.

Regardless of the pricing of gametes on the basis of the donors' traits and qualifications, there is something unnerving about the way recipients project their norms and beliefs regarding the "ideal child" (and, *eo ipso*, the "ideal human being") onto the reproductive materials. Martin's (2014) study of the American donor industry reveals an industry flagrantly based on racial and elitist ideologies wherein would-be parents are what one informant, a "donor broker" named Megan referred to as "freakishly picky" when selecting their donors. First of all, the recipients of reproductive materials wanted "somebody who's bright," Megan said (cited in Martin, 2014: 439): In addition, Megan claimed, "[W]e work with a lot of models and actresses, and they get chosen all the time. So basically, *we look for candidates that people would really choose.*" "Kind of the creepy thing about egg donation is that a lot of people will just choose a beautiful donor," Megan claimed (cited in Martin, 2014: 440). Megan was also concerned that what she described as "the 'slippery slope' from PDG" to the "'genetically engineering a baby to look just the way they [recipient clients] want,'" were permitted and even encouraged in the industry. Megan questioned whether the would-be parents were really going to "love their children less because they have green eyes, or brown eyes?," and thus regarded this "crazy" behavior as something that "seemed really Nazi" to her (cited in Martin, 2014: 440).

Finally, Martin (2014) shows that the clients of donor brokers tended to assume that donor traits would of necessity be passed down to the offspring, as if reproductive material was some kind of vending machine purchase: "Couples sometimes demanded that donors have blue eyes and a certain type of nose, for example or refused any donor that had acne or braces as a child" (Martin, 2014: 446). In Martin's view, one can here speak about a conversation or translation of *cultural capital* into *genetic capital* as some kind of mechanical procedure:

Demand for donors with advanced degrees, musical ability, and Ivy League pedigrees, implies that these markers of class and rearing are genetically transmissible; cultural capital is thus a manifestation of, and shorthand for, genetic capital. Egg donor's genetic capital becomes a marketable commodity, with their cultural capital as convenient shorthand.

(Martin, 2014: 440)

The recipients of ova and sperm thus worked hard to ensure that their investment in the baby-to-come maximized their utility in terms of future cultural capital. Hopefully, in the next stage, economic and financial capital would be generated on the basis of this stock of genetic and cultural capital.

Critics of gametes markets and trade, especially the international trade, are concerned about the exploitation of female donors in particular, and frown at the idea of "gift giving" as an all too rosy ideological construct that conceals the true motive of these donors, derived from their inability to support themselves and their families unless they enact themselves as a reservoir of attractive reproductive materials. For instance, Caucasian women in Ukraine or Russia are paid as little as one fifth of the price paid by clients in IVF clinics in Cyprus (Dickenson, 2008: 6), an evidence of economic compensation being so low that it borders on exploitation on the part of these clinics. These egg donors are thus better termed "egg sellers" than donors, both Dickenson (2008: 5) and Twine (2011) argue: "The term egg and sperm donations are misnomers since individuals are not donating their eggs or sperm in an act of altruism, but selling them for a price" (Twine, 2011: 32).

Despite these concerns and conditions reported, not all gamete markets are of necessity based on exploitative and unethical practices. Almeling's (2011, 2007) study of egg and sperm donors in California, one of the states with the most liberal legislation for the use of ART, and also permitting surrogacy, shows how various social and cultural beliefs and norms intersect in the trade of gametes. First of all, while male donors have to demonstrate adequate sperm quality, measured in terms of sperm concentration and sperm motility and otherwise being healthy, the female donors were expected by the egg agency staff to "conform to one or two gendered stereotypes:" To be either "highly educated and physically attractive" – a sporty and good-looking, preferably tall, Ivy league student would be the perfect match for the agency – or be "caring and motherly with children of her own," a set of qualities that underline the desired norm of empathy and concern for family life being in harmony with the gift-giving ideology that the egg agencies actively promoted (Almeling, 2007: 327).

In addition, while sperm donation was surrounded by various forms of joking, in themselves quite harmless and possibly serving the role to mediate the tensions created when being expected to masturbate in a clinical setting, the female donors were expected to have a less lighthearted relationship to their eggs. "[W]omen are perceived as more closely connected to their eggs than men are to their sperm," Almeling (2007: 328) stresses. For instance, female donors were from the very beginning encouraged to think of themselves not so much as being part of a faceless market transaction similar to that of buying an insurance or a bag of groceries but to be part of a "gift relationship" with the recipients: "[E]gg agencies structure the exchange not only as a legalistic economic transaction, but also the beginning of a caring gift cycle, which the staff fosters by expressing appreciation to the donors, both on behalf of the agency and the agency's clients" (Almeling, 2007: 333).

One of the consequences of this seemingly odd combination of profit motive on the part of both the egg agency and the donor and the gift-giving ideology was that the female donors were prevented from thinking of what they were doing as a "job" or even as a "career choice." Instead, they were encouraged to think of themselves as participating in the amazing female prerogative to "help others" by "giving the gift of life" (Almeling, 2007: 334): "[W]omen who attempted to make a career of selling eggs provoke disgust among staff, in part because they violate the altruistic framing of donation" (ibid.). This inclusion in gift relationships was further underlined by the custom of the recipients to give the female donors flowers, jewelry, or an additional financial gift in addition to the formal compensation, a practice that served the role of "[u]pholding the constructed vision of egg donation as reciprocal gift-giving, in which egg donors help recipients and recipients help donors" (ibid.). In Almeling's account, such practices both draw on and reproduce stereotypes of women as being "selfless, caring, and focused on relationships and family" (Almeling, 2011: 131).

Female donors also occasionally received pictures and letters from the recipients after the birth of the baby, something that few if any sperm donors reported. These differences represent both gendered stereotypes but also how the sperm banks organized their activities and how they encouraged their donors to think of what they were doing precisely as professional work that needs to be conducted with care and skill in order to produce "passable samples" (Almeling, 2011: 131). In this way, sperm donors were subject to less social and normative control as long as their sperm samples passed the quality checks.

Somewhat paradoxically, the female donors that were actively encouraged to think of themselves as being part of a social relation and giving the gift of life, did not think of themselves as being the mother of these children. In contrast, the male donors both discussed and joked about having "many children" while not speaking of their own families. In brief, male donors depicted themselves as "fathers" while female donors were "not-mothers" (Almeling, 2011: 145–165). Almeling again makes reference to social and cultural norms, where men's connections between the gametes and fatherhood can be expressed as the straightforward connection Sperm→Baby. In the case of women, the enactment of motherhood involves a longer sequence of biological and social and cultural processes, formalized by Almeling as follows: Eggs→Fertilization→Implantation→Pregnancy→Birth→ Child rearing. That is, to be a father, it is enough to contribute with a sperm sample, while motherhood includes a long series of reproductive, gestational, and nurturing activities and undertakings over a longer period of time, excluding the egg donor from claims of motherhood proper.

These differences between male and female donors also translated into how they addressed their financial motives. While the male donors were a little concerned about speaking about their remuneration as a "salary" or "pay," Almeling (2011) says that the female donors were more prone to speak of "compensation" – a term that implies a loss or something unfulfilled. Female donors had to undergo further ordeal to give their "gift of life" than the male donors, and their gametes are also more limited, two conditions that underlined their sense of loss regardless of the more than 40 times higher economic compensation. This attitude is also aligned with the general prohibition enforced by egg agencies staff to think of egg donation as a job.

Taken together, regardless of the rosy gift of life ideology being actively promoted and enforced, by the end of the day, Almeling (2011) argues, it was economic incentives and financial motivations that dominated the trade of gametes. Therefore, the trade of gametes is no proper gift economy, nor is it a typical market in the conventional sense of the term, neutrally connecting sellers and buyers. Instead, the market for gametes is characterized by its idiosyncratic combination of social, cultural, economic, and regulatory conditions that need to be kept in balance and mutually adjusted. Not least the market for gametes and the actors involved are concerned about the social legitimacy of how human reproductive materials become subject to financial and economic interests, a condition that violated the taboo against blending money and intimacy (Zelizer, 2005).

The run-of-the-mill practice: in vitro fertilization

Of the various ART and therapies derived from reproductive medicine research, in vitro fertilization (or IVF, for short), remains the mainstream and least controversial. IVF has been practiced since the end of the 1970s, and there is today an extensive scientific literature reporting clinical studies demonstrating that IVF is a safe and relatively efficient therapy (roughly 50 percent of all patients succeed in becoming parents) that has helped hundreds of thousands of sub-fertile couples and single women become parents. Regardless of the medical and clinical success of IVF, there are still debates and controversies around who should be eligible for the therapy and who should carry the costs for the therapy.

For instance, in Longino's (1992: 326) critical accounts, IVF is treated as a resource in disciplining populations through political decisions regarding what social groups are qualified for the therapy. As a consequence, IVF serves to performatively reproduce ideas about females and their role in society: "Access to in vitro fertilization is more widely restricted to those who fit what have been thought to be appropriate criteria for motherhood: heterosexuality, marriage, absence of disabilities. These patterns of restriction and access reinforce traditional conceptions of women's place in society." Other commentators such as Franklin (1998) point at how biomedical technologies serve to reduce components and processes of human reproduction to discrete events and occurrences that in turn can be handled separately. Franklin (ibid.: 104) illustrates with the case of the separation between conception and fertilization. Previously being synonymous as being part of the "natural conception" of the oocyte, but now *fertilization* is defined as the fusion of gametes (the egg and sperm), while *conception* is "[t]he process of genetic combination, which occurs over the succeeding thirty-six hours," in the process *embryogenesis* (ibid.: 106).

Critique of the reductionist qualities of IVF is also highlighted by Cussins' (1998, 1996) ethnographic study of IVF practices in the clinic and Becker's (2000) study of IVF patients. Anne-Marie Mol (2002) speaks of the "body multiple" in medical clinical practice, the decomposing of the human body into distinct and separated domains of professional expertise and jurisdictional claims, and Becker (2000: 26) addresses what she claims is a "common problem" in assisted reproduction, the feeling of being "de-personalized" and seeing oneself as "an assemblage of body parts" to be examined separately. Cussins (1998, 1996) regards the treatment of the female reproductive apparatus in similar reductionist terms. Using the term "ontological choreography" to discuss how various reproductive capacities and reproductive materials are over time isolated, combined, and reunited, Cussins (1996) speaks of two processes in IVF therapy: *naturalization* and *bureaucratization*.

Naturalization here denotes the process in which humans are transformed into "objects of experimentation and manipulation," while bureaucratization is the extensive legislative and bureaucratic standard operation procedures and routines that structure the clinical work, e.g., the keeping of extensive statistical records in the clinic. These two processes serve to render the IVF patient an ensemble of "mechanistic discrete body parts" subject to manipulation. The bureaucratization process is in turn embedded in a particular epistemic culture that in many ways encourages and feeds on the "production of statistics," Cussins (1998: 85) argues: "Fertility clinics, particularly private ones, are increasingly in competition for patients. Reputation draw patients, and these are built primarily on the rate of successful pregnancies. A patient calling an infertility unit has a right to, and often will, ask what the center's success rates are." As a consequence, much energy goes into "compiling the statistics and generating success rates." In addition, "competitors' rates are viewed with interest and sometimes with suspicion, and ways in which reported rates from center to center might not be comparable are much discussed" (ibid.).

Cussins (1998, 1996) provides a first-hand account of the work conducted in IVF clinics, and it demands no extraordinary degrees of empathy on part of the reader to see how it can be stressful to undergo IVF therapies. As Franklin (2013: 7) remarks, "in vitro fertilization is not a simple process of steps leading to potential success – it is a confusing and stressful world of disjointed temporalities, jangled emotions, difficult decisions, unfamiliar procedures, medical jargon, and metabolic chaos." At the same time, most health care therapies are of necessity stressful for the patient, and regardless of Cussins' evocative theorizing, her study does not counteract the fact that there is a substantial demand for IVF therapies regardless of the female patient's sense of vulnerability and the actual risks involved in e.g., the hormone therapies that precede the egg retrieval. In this perspective, Cussins' (1998, 1996) seminal work is indicative of feminist theory-informed accounts of IVF as being in its essence exploitative and representing an instrumental application of technoscientific know-how and tools and machinery.

Another set of criticism pertaining to IVF therapies addresses how clinics tend to underrate the failure rates and the efforts needed on the part of the female patients – a trait this industry shares with the cosmetic surgery industry that also presents, critics claim, a positive and affirmative account of the services offered (see e.g., Pitts-Taylor, 2007). Franklin emphasizes this aspect:

> The tantalizing feature of IVF is the idea that there *is* just a minor adjustment to be made, just a small gap to be bridged, just a little push in the right direction, just the need for a 'helping hand,' as the technique is often described. More often than not, several adjustments are needed, and consequently there is a significant component of trial and error in identifying them.
>
> (Franklin, 1998: 109)

In contrast, as the studies reveal, many patients find the therapy emotionally exhausting, the hormone therapies very stressful and occasionally leading to hospitalization, and the egg retrieval painful, and by the end of the day, every second sub-fertile couple or single women leave the clinics disappointed as they have failed to become pregnant despite all the efforts and costs. At the same time, there are regulatory agencies and policy-making bodies that monitor the industry and the legal frameworks that determine the activities in the clinics are constantly moderated to accommodate the most recent clinical research findings. For instance, in the early days of IVF practices, when more than one embryo was selected and returned to the uterus, there were "above the natural average" twin births among assisted reproduction babies. Around 25 percent of all IVF babies had low birth weight and spent time in intensive care (Rapp, 2011: 207). Later on, it was found that "these children are bound for special education at disproportionately high rates" (Rapp, 2011: 207). Pfeffer adds:

> During the 1980s, as a result of assisted conception technology, the number of triplets, quins, and quads born increased by almost 50 percent. However, women with a higher-order multiple pregnancy are more likely to experience complications and have a more difficult labor, and their babies have a higher chance of being born prematurely and of having health problems demanding intensive medical care, as well as putting considerable pressure on special care bay units.
>
> (Pfeffer, 1999: 170)

However, as clinical research studies revealed these conditions, clinical practices changed in countries like Sweden and eventually the legislation prohibited multiple embryo transfers. "After legislation declaring that only a single embryo could be implanted via IVF, Sweden saw its NICU [Neonatal Intensive Care Unit] usage rates plummet, as did Belgium, and now much of the European Union has followed suit" (Rapp, 2011: 211, note 7). However, still today in regulated markets like the U.S., multiple embryo transfers are widespread in private clinics, serving patients that pay for their therapies themselves. Swedish clinicians and reproductive medicine researchers regard such clinical practices as an appalling violation of the medical principle *primum non nocere* – "first, do no harm" – but it is a risk taken in order to maximize the chances of conceiving a child. Apparently, U.S. regulatory bodies regard the clinical studies that point at the risk with multiple embryo transfers differently than their European counterparts.

Controversial practices: surrogacy

Surrogacy is based on in vitro fertilization therapies and enables a woman to serve as the so-called gestational surrogacy mother receiving an embryo fertilized in the laboratory. In the literature, there is a distinction made between *full surrogacy* wherein the surrogate mother carries a fetus where the oocyte is her own, and *gestational surrogacy* wherein both the egg and the sperm are donated by others. In either case, surrogacy is treated as what is in various ways morally questionable and what is potentially exploiting the woman carrying the fetus, or otherwise violating norms of human dignity. These various moral views and considerations are reflected in the diverse legal frameworks being enacted in various countries and states in e.g., the U.S. Twine (2011) makes a connection between gestational surrogacy and "transnational capitalist markets" where various power relations determine the supply and demand and the pricing of not only reproductive materials and reproductive services but all sorts of biological tissues and resources:

> Gestational surrogacy is embedded in a transnational capitalist market that is structured by racial, ethnic, and class inequalities and by competing nation-state regulatory regimes ... There is unequal access to assisted reproduction technologies in most countries because the cost is prohibitive and if it is not state funded then only elites and the upper middle classes can afford to purchase these services.
>
> (Twine, 2011: 3)

For Twine (2011), gestational surrogacy is a privilege for the financially favored classes, and consequently economic inequality lies at the very heart of the surrogacy arrangement. Despite such concerns, the market for surrogacy services has grown sharply over the last few years, Mohapatra (2012: 413) reports: "Despite many countries' prohibitions or restrictions on surrogacy arrangements, the market for international surrogacy has grown to an estimated size of six billion dollars annually worldwide." For instance, in India, surrogacy services are today a million-dollar business:

> Surrogacy is estimated to be a $445 million business in India ... The Confederation of Indian Industry predicts that medical tourism, including surrogacy, could generate $2,3 billion in annual revenue by 2012. Gestational surrogacy is an important gendered niche in the global medical market.
>
> (Twine, 2011: 17)

In 2009, India had 350 facilities that offered surrogacy as part of a broader array of infertility-treatment services, three times as many as in 2005. These clinics reported approximately 1,500 pregnancy attempts using surrogates in 2009 (Mohapatra, 2012: 433). The costs and the prices for surrogacy services also reflect regional differences in "production factor prices," where e.g., the costs in the U.S. are much higher than in e.g., Ukraine and India. "The typical costs for a surrogacy arrangement in the United States ranges from $80,000 and $120,000, of which the surrogate receives between $14,000 and $18,000," Mohapatra (ibid.: 428) writes. In Ukraine, a popular country for surrogacy services because of lenient regulations and a supply of women with the same phenotype as many of the Western couples that can afford surrogacy services, a "surrogacy arrangement costs approximately '$30,000 to $45,000 for foreign parents' whereof $10,000 to $15,000 'going to the surrogate mother'" (ibid.: 431). Finally, in India the costs are around $12,000 – a fraction of the costs in the United States – whereof the surrogate earns between $2,500 and $7,000 (ibid.: 435).

The exploitation of poor and uneducated women in e.g., India is a standing concern in the surrogacy literature, but in fact the payment a surrogate receives for carrying a fetus is in many cases four to five times their annual household income (Mohapatra, 2012: 436). This significant income does not in any way justify surrogacy per se, but primarily indicates the enormous differences in income between ethnic groups, social classes, and regions. In the U.S., it is often working class women, housewives and home-makers, and not infrequently so-called "army-wives," women married to military workers and located close to army bases where there are limited work opportunities, who serve as surrogates. American surrogacy is thus determined by class relations and the work opportunities of American working class women:

> [Surrogates] are typically working-class women who, by receiving remuneration for what are essentially devalued homemaking skills in American culture, elevate their gender status by becoming professional homemakers. As professional homemakers, they receive the attentions of wealthier middle-to-upper class couples and are celebrated at their surrogate centers as commendable altruists.
>
> (Goslinga-Roy, 2000: 133)

The concept of altruism (to be discussed in more detail shortly) is here the key to the industry. Rather that treating surrogacy services as legitimate work and a source of income, altruism is a term that effectively serves to conceal the reification and commodification of reproductive capacities. Similar to Almeling's (2007) study of egg donors, participation in the reproduction industry cannot be treated as regular work but needs to be understood as a form of gift giving regardless of the economic transactions the exchange of gift entails.

As Mohapatra (2012: 414) points out, despite the strong evidence of acute risks of exploiting poor and uneducated, mostly rural women in e.g., India, the Western press has generated "mostly positive reports about success stories in international surrogacy." Just because infertility and childlessness are topics that everyone easily can feel a great deal of sympathy for the darker sides of the surrogacy business are frequently ignored. Activists working in the industry are often portrayed as the servants of despairing and unhappy couples, and the financial interests and transactions involved are at times downplayed. At the same time, there are many alarming stories reported in both news media and in legal cases that reveal practices that many would find appalling or morally questioning. For instance, Mohapatra (2012: 415) accounts for the case of how Theresa Erickson and Hillary Neiman, two "well-known surrogacy attorneys" in California, and Carla Chambers, a "six-time surrogate," hired Ukraine surrogate mothers for a cost of $38,000–45,000 per surrogate to create their own "baby-factory" facilities:

> At the time these embryos were implanted and the months afterwards, these 'surrogates' carried fetuses for which there were no intended parents of surrogacy agreements. Instead Erickson, Chambers, and Neiman waited until the women were in their second trimester of pregnancy, when the chance of miscarriage was smaller…
>
> (Mohapatra, 2012: 416–417)

After the first trimester, the attorneys advertised to potential adoptive parents that a "Caucasian" infant was available due to a surrogacy arrangement that "fell through": "This arrangement led to the placement of at least a dozen babies, and potential adoptive parents paid from $100,000 to $150,000 to assume the supposed surrogacy arrangement" (Mohapatra, 2012: 416–417).

Ukraine was here selected on the basis of the lenient legal and regulatory framework for IVF and surrogacy and because of the good supply of surrogates, and thereafter American couples were invited to "adopt a fetus," a baby not yet born but still in the womb. In another case, a French couple engaged a Ukrainian surrogate that gave birth to twins, but as surrogacy is illegal in France, the babies were not recognized by the state of France. In addition, under Ukrainian law the twins were French because the legal parents were French. This controversy made the babies "effectively stateless" (Mohapatra, 2012: 421). Such legal inconsistencies is a standing concern in, for instance, the U.S., hosting a sprawling surrogacy industry where over recent years, gestational surrogacy rates have risen almost 400 percent and today around 1,400 babies are now born in the United States annually (ibid.: 424). Despite this growth in supply and demand, each state maintains its own legislation. In Wisconsin, there is in fact no legislation at all regarding surrogacy, leaving the issue of whether "[s]urrogacy agreements will be enforced in the event of a conflict an open question" (ibid.: 428). In international law, there are just as many differences between countries and regions, with quite generous surrogacy legislation in e.g., Israel and a legal ban in many countries and with a number of countries in-between, permitting what has been called *altruistic surrogacy*.

The concept of altruism has been heavily debated in the health care policy and bioethics literature, and today there is an agreement among scholars that altruism:

"(1) seeks to increase another's welfare, not one's own; (2) is voluntary; (3) is intentional, meant to help someone else; and (4) expects no external rewards" (Healy, 2004: 388). Healy (ibid.: 391), studying organ donation rather than surrogacy, still believes that there is a need to shift from "social-psychological explanations" of altruism to "institutional sources of individual actions and identities." That is, the decision to act altruistically or not is less the effect of personal convictions and beliefs as it is "[s]tructured, promoted, and made logistically possible by organizations and institutions with a strong interest in producing it," i.e., altruism is "highly institutionalized" (ibid.: 387). In this view, policy-makers decisions and activities regarding e.g., the legalization of surrogacy signaling that surrogacy is a socially legitimate practice that may be encouraged can influence individuals' decisions to act altruistically. Expressed differently, the institutional and socio-cultural setting wherein surrogacy decisions are made can make a difference.

For example, one of the key concerns for scholars studying the surrogacy industry in India is that participation in these activities is highly stigmatizing for the women, and in many cases, poorly educated rural women do not fully understand the clinical procedures they are expected to undergo, making the legal concept of "consent" troublesome (Pande, 2010, 2009). In order to not exploit these women, there are today discussions about legalizing. In such cases, the risks of exploitation would in the ideal case be lower and the economic and financial gains would only play a more marginal role than in the case of the Indian commercial surrogacy. In e.g., Sweden, this discussion (to be accounted for in the empirical part of this volume) has to date not led to a more lenient view of surrogacy as altruistic surrogacy is expected to serve only as a complement to commercial services and would possibly even further legitimize the pay-for-services arrangements offered in India and elsewhere. That is, altruistic behavior and the juridical recognition of such acts serve to expand the possibilities for *all kinds* of surrogacy. Unintended consequences of purposeful action are therefore anticipated to avoid the exploitation of women.

Studies of surrogacy

The legal, regulatory, and ethical concerns regarding surrogacy are substantial and the literature is significant, but there is also a literature reporting empirical studies of surrogacy work. This literature reports studies of surrogates in Western countries such as in Israel (Teman, 2010) and the U.S. (Snowdon, 1994), or examines overseas industries in e.g., India (Pande, 2010, 2009). Teman (2010) presents ethnographic work conducted in Israel, a country with the most liberal legalization in the world, which actively encourages surrogacy. In Teman's account, there are no pressing ethical issues that would undermine the legitimacy of surrogacy, but rather the narrative focuses on how the surrogates need to develop strategies and tactics for distancing themselves from the parents that both care for the surrogate's well-being and health but also may be opinionated about the everyday life of the surrogate mothers. Teman's (2010) research thus provides a valuable insight into an institutional setting wherein surrogacy is effectively institutionalized, but possibly also reflects these shared norms and beliefs of the Israeli community. Snowdon (1994) presents interview data with women that participate in egg donation and surrogacy, and she stresses how these women have a strong sense of participating in a gift economy where they can help sub-fertile couples becoming parents. Also Snowdon's study presents no major objections against surrogacy per se, as it is ultimately based on the unforced participation of women that demonstrate a great deal of sympathy for couples suffering from their inability to become parents.

Pande's (2010, 2009) seminal fieldwork collected in the Indian surrogacy industry presents an entirely different story, not so much of mutual interests and shared concerns across the surrogate parents' boundary as it stresses the immediate financial benefits of Indian surrogates but also the costs this work induces. In Pande's account, the women participating in surrogacy do this "clinical labor" because it generates substantial incomes and the concepts of gift-giving and gift-economies seem to be less pronounced than in the Israeli and U.S. cases – in fact, such ideas seem quite alien to the local industry. In addition, the Indian women strongly believe they are entitled to their economic compensation on the basis of their efforts, and in many cases the clinics (e.g., the well-known clinic in Anand, Gujarat) help the women open their own bank accounts to ensure that the women themselves, not their husbands or brothers, can access the money. Pande also emphasizes the importance of the institutional and clinical setting, capable of transforming – very much like in any form of management of labor – the poor and by and large uneducated rural women into "perfect surrogates" and perfect "clinical laborers" – "cheap, docile, selfless, and nurturing" (Pande, 2010: 970).

Fertility clinics and "surrogacy hostels" are therefore the sites wherein surrogacy is assembled into clinical services and accompanying clinical labor. In Pande's account, these activities represent a "disciplinary process" where the Indian women become "perfect mother-workers for national and international clients" (Pande, 2010: 970). Pande thus effectively undermines the predominant image of surrogacy as a form of advanced gift-giving and instead stresses the industrial and managerial features of the industry, by and large similar to any other industrial service production, including new forms of labor that are embedded in a variety of legal and institutional conditions and the access to technoscientific and clinical know-how and resources (ibid.: 972). In shifting the focus from the romantic and therefore highly appealing narrative of surrogacy as a social exchange of gifts on the basis of a blend of altruistic sentiments and (playing only a secondary role in the exchange relationship) economic transactions to a more straightforward and therefore also more credible view, underlining the clinical labor of the surrogates, Pande (ibid.) serves to demystify the industry. Rather than being concealed by a rosy haze of joint commitment to procreation, surrogacy is a business venture where financial resources exchange hands to provide clinical labor that cannot be offered elsewhere. For Pande (ibid.) the gift-giving ideology is a flattering but emotionally and culturally useful resource for the industry. In other words, it must not prevent analysts from recognizing the institutional and financial arrangements that constitute the industry. "For Pande," Bailey (2011: 724–725) comments, "surrogate motherhood is not a moral dilemma to be solved; it is a structural reality to be understood. Contract pregnancy is neither moral nor immoral, neither virtuous nor vicious; it is simply the way things are for many Indian women." In addition, Bailey (ibid.: 726) proposes, this strategic reduction of the element of intimacy in the trade may help Indian women participating in the industry reduce their stigmata: "Redefining surrogacy work as sexualized care labor is a sensible step towards reducing the stigmatized harms associated with surrogacy work."

In summary, studies of surrogacy conducted in the Western part of the world stresses the altruistic elements of the clinical labor, and studies of e.g., the Indian surrogacy industry stress the economic and financial rationale of the participants, not only the surrogates but also the clinic owners and the (Western) clients. While this research reveals few activities and conditions that would undermine the credibility of the industry, it also points at the various ethical, moral, and practical issues that need to be carefully negotiated and constantly reflected upon, especially in the Indian case. In other words, the empirical studies neither confirm, nor eliminate the arguments for or against surrogacy being addressed in legal and policy-making quarters.

Assisted reproductive technologies in the making

One of the great paradoxes of the contemporary period is that the more the biomedical technosciences have advanced and the better therapies and treatments that are being offered, the more people tend to mistrust the sciences and remain skeptical regarding their "intervening into nature" (Habermas, 2003). "Seldom has the future of human nature been the subject of such concerns and in-depth discussions by our wise public intellectuals as in our globalized age," Braidotti, (2008: 10) writes. In Braidotti's (2008) view, such "technophobic reactions to our bio-technological progress" has created the possibilities for a return to what she calls a "Kantian moral universalism" prescribing what can be legitimately conducted and what cannot.

At the same time, there is much hope and hype around the biomedical technosciences, leading to what Brown and Michael (2003) speak of as a "sociology of expectations," the scholarly pursuit to understand how professional and lay communities jointly create expectations around the new scientific wonders that are in the making and how these new possibilities will affect everyday life. For instance, in popular news media, it is commonplace that medicine researchers present research findings and make the standard prediction that "in ten years' time, there may be a proper therapy." In many cases, such predictions are vastly underestimating the time needed to bring new therapies to the market, leading to these statements being less credible, yet reproducing social expectations regarding what the biomedical technosciences are capable of accomplishing. In this section, a few promising fields in the intersection between reproductive medicine and e.g., stem cell therapies and regenerative medicine now being part of the biomedical technosciences will be examined. Some of these novel concepts and therapies, including uterus transplantation, are quite spectacular and certainly pushed the boundaries for ART and the biomedical technosciences more broadly.

Preimplantation genomics diagnosis and screening (PGD and PGS)

One of the novel concepts being used in e.g., IVF therapies but also being more widely recognized as a promising method for the future is what is called *preimplantation genetic diagnosis* (PGD) and *preimplantation genetic screening* (PGS). These two diagnostic methods are used to identify genetic sequences that signify diseases such as Huntington's disease, Down's syndrome, or other disorders derived from damages to the genetic code. The very idea of the human genome as being a form of "script" or "code" underlying human life represents a major shift in biology from the examination of the *phenotype* of organisms, their physical features and the organs and tissue, to the *genotype*, the molecular structure of biological organisms. Warren Weaver, perhaps most well-known for his ground-breaking work on the mathematical theory of information in collaboration with Claude Shannon, coined the term *molecular biology* in 1938 (Kay, 2000: 45). In 1944, the great Austrian physicist Erwin Schrödinger published a book entitled *What is Life?*, wherein he proposed that all forms of life were based on a "code-script" that could lend itself to scholarly analysis. This shift from the organ and cellular level to the molecular level of the organism helped biology stop being what Neville Symonds (cited in Kay, 2000: 61) referred to as a "sissy subject" and "came of age." As Black (2014) and many other commentators make clear, in this new orientation of biology – a "white coat biology" rather than the "green biology" of the past – the concept of information plays a decisive role. In the Western episteme, the Aristotelian distinction between form and matter and the idea that they could not be reduced to one another has structured human thinking (Black, 2014: 118), but in the "age of information," the concept of information serves precisely the role of collapsing these two terms into one single entity:

> Acting on matter at a molecular scale produces the idea that *matter itself is a code*: atoms are a fixed, finite and predictable set of components that gives rise to all matter simply through the variation in their arrangement.
>
> (Black, 2014: 118. Emphasis added)

From this perspective, all types of matter and objects have the same building blocks, just differently combined: "[M]y heart, a lead, a spiderweb and a diamond are all composed of the same carbon atoms; the only difference is their syntax – the way in which these carbon atoms are arranged and combined" (Black, 2014: 118).

The nanotechnology discourse, for instance, rests on this idea, that matter can be "re-coded" and suddenly in this science fiction scenario, one category of matter can be transformed into another structure (Choi and Mody, 2009; Bensaude-Vincent,

2007; Berube, 2006; Milburn, 2005). As a consequence, information is "everywhere" and everything can be both presented and manipulated as "information structures" (Thomas and Acuña-Narvaez, 2006; Jones, 2004): "The informatics account has conquered every possible territory," Black (2014: 119) argues.

In the biomedical technosciences, the development of information-based scientific concepts such as genomics and proteomics, rests on such post-Aristotelian ideas where form and matter is nothing more than the expression of their informational content. The concept of genomics and specific research programs such as HUGO, the human genome mapping project in the 1990s attracted significant media attention, and spokespersons frequently told stories about the human genome as being the "book of life" and assured that as soon as the mapping of the human genome was finished, therapies for a range of illnesses and medical conditions would follow suit (Lock, 2007: 62). "A complete set of genes, the genome, carries instructions, or a blueprint, for the development and function of an entire organism," Zweiger (2001: 16) claims, testifying to the enthusiastic reception of genomics. Critics, in turn, spoke more neutrally of a "genocentric biology" (Griesemer, 2006: 210) or more explicitly about the unwarranted expectations laid upon the ability to decode the genome's operative functioning (Sunder Rajan, 2006).

Today, two decades after the human genome mapping project, researchers are less sure about the "book of life" view of the human genome. "The genome sequence has a far greater capacity to mislead than it has to illuminate," Higgs, 2004 (cited in Hopkins et al., 2007: 583) says. "Today, we are told that the age of the genome is past, that the genome no longer provides all the answers, that we have instead Rnomics (for RNA), proteomics, systeomics, and physiomics," Fujimura (2005: 197) adds. The principal hypothesis of genomics, that there is a one-way path from DNA to RNA to proteins, "can no longer be sustained," Rose (2007: 47) claims. As a consequence of these new research findings regarding the immense complexity of biological organisms, researchers today speak of the "post-genomic era" as the period where researchers no longer believe in one single informational structure, that of the DNA and the human genome, but rather examine the complex *interactions* between single genes, so-called Single Nucleotide Polymorphisms (SNPs, commonly pronounced "snipps." Rajan, 2006: 50), RNA, and the proteins being generated. "By 'post-genomic' I mean the recognition, since the 2001 mapping of the human genome, that there were too few genes to explain whole-organism traits in simple genetic determinist terms," Wynne (2005: 87, note 2) writes.

While the mapping of the human genome did not reveal all the secrets of life, this by no means suggests that this new know-how was not practically useful in both the biomedical technosciences and in clinical practices. Kohli-Laven et al. (2011) examine the implications from using genomic techniques to prescribe therapies for cancer patients, opening up for what at times are, perhaps euphemistically, referred to as *personalized medicine* – individually adjusted therapies depending on a series of biological traits. In addition, Lemke (2011: 94) discusses what he calls *genetic engineering* as a research program based on a "political epistemology of life" that no longer deals with the "control of external nature but rather the transformation of inner nature." In many cases, the identification of particular gene sequences, e.g., the BRCA1 gene sequence correlating with breast cancer, can help anticipate illnesses and to identify target groups. However, while these new biomedical concepts and therapies may prolong and improve the quality of life, the very process of genetic categorization is not devoid of difficulties (Latimer et al., 2006: 600). In Latimer et al.'s (ibid.: 601) account, genetic diagnosis is riddled by ambivalence and uncertainty as the clinical work always includes "categorical work" that has "as much to do with the construction and refinement of categories as with their mere application" (ibid.: 601). That is, in clinical work in dysmorphology, the categories used are both the vehicle and the outcome from the work as categories are created *en route*. Genetic diagnosis is therefore always at risk of being based on theories that are not yet able to prove their therapeutic accuracy.

In the field of reproductive medicine and ART, genomics methods have been used for quite some time to identify genetic sequences that correlate with certain medical conditions. PGD and PGS are today both widely used in clinical practice and a candidate for being a technology that could be given a larger role in ART. Spar (2010: 184) straightforwardly speaks of PGD as a "[p]athbreaking technology that allows parents to select an embryo with particular genetic characteristics," indicating the laboratory benefits of the technology. In contrast, a number of commentators have expressed their concerns regarding the use of PGD and PGS to create "designer babies," to abort fetuses with undesirable traits on the basis of either efficiency criteria or preconceived ideas about what are desirable and attractive human qualities. An unrestricted use of such technologies would thus reduce the barriers between being "born and made" (in Franklin and Roberts' [2006] apt formulation). Goodwin (2011: 843) thus suggests that PGD represents "[t]he maximization of choice in the ART realm." Such arguments indicate that ART are at risk to establish a form of "free to choose" market wherein parents could preorder personality characteristics and traits from a menu – evidence from the gamete market suggests it is "human" to think in such terms, favoring "nature" over "nurture" (Keller, 2010) – and where any deviation from some prescribed "standard baby" would be treated as "odd choices." As a consequence of these controversies, the international legislation is quite diverse: "Some countries ban PGD outright, others regulate the use as a means to screen for chromosomal abnormalities, allow PGD only to screen for specific diseases, or prohibits its use for sex-selective purpose" (Martin, 2014: 436).

Fortunately, such an "eugenic medicine" scenario is complicated to accomplish, less skeptical commentators such as Robertson (2010: 200) argue: "The fear that embryo screening will lead to a market in genetically engineered children available only to the wealthy is overblown. Wanting a healthy child is natural, and we already have a well-established system of prenatal screening for many anomalies." In addition, Robertson (2010: 201) assures, this fear of babies "being made" on industrial basis through the aid of PGD and PGS would demand substantially more detailed knowledge regarding the intricate relations between various genetic material and their translations into proteins and how these molecular processes translate into phenotypes and social traits. "We simply do not know enough about the genomics of desirable traits to subject them to embryo screening in what that would attract people not otherwise undergoing IVF," Robertson (ibid.) writes.

At the same time, as will be indicated in Part II of this volume, an expanded use of PGD and PGS would possibly be helpful for couples and single women that fail to become pregnant despite their embryos looking qualified and otherwise appearing to follow the regular development pattern. In these cases, new ways to make use of genomics analysis would be helpful in identifying if there are any genetic variations in the embryos that can explain the infertility. An expanded use of PGD and PGS would thus advance genomics analyses, which in turn would serve to increasingly treat embryos as carriers of hereditary material that may lend itself to biomedical technoscientific analysis and choices on the basis of such practices. Needless to say, this is not an uncontroversial scenario for all stakeholders.

From the molecular to the organ level: uterus transplantation and the role of transplant surgery

In addition to the more conventional ART and the development of practices that increase the precision of existing therapies, there are some examples of how reproductive medicine in obstetrics and gynecology are combined with organ transplant surgery. Organ transplant surgery is today a widespread domain of expertise and there is a strictly regulated market of human organs (Sharp, 2007, 2003; Lock, 2002). Needless to say, unlike the case of children, embryos, and human gametes, there are few serious commentators that have advocated free-market solutions to the endemic global organ supply shortage as that would open up for a large share of the human population as being worth more dead than alive; for instance, while there are rumors that kidneys and livers are traded illegally for hundreds of thousands of dollars, many human beings live on less than a dollar a day, testifying to how humans are valued in the globalized economy. As a consequence, there are rumors circulating in poor communities in e.g., the slums of the metropolitan areas in the developing world, that organ theft is part of organized crime, but there is still little evidence of such activities (Das, 2000). Yet, the persistency of this rumor testifies to the "externalities" such "organ markets" would create (see e.g., Cherry, 2005).

As reported in Part II of this volume, there is ongoing scientific research work that tries to transplant a womb from a donor to a recipient in order to help women born without ovaries to become mothers. In the case of the patients involved in the research program in Sweden, it is mostly mothers agreeing to transfer their uterus to their daughter in an attempt to examine whether this could be one approach to create reproductive capacities. In many cases these research programs have been approached with skepticism, not because they would violate any moral or normative beliefs regarding human reproduction as the surgery skills are based on widespread organ transplant surgery procedures but because they consume time, energy, research skills, and money that could be allocated differently. That is, as in numerous other cases, reproductive medicine is surrounded by the idea that infertility is not really a medical condition legitimately subject to medical treatment and research but should be tolerated as a fact, perhaps even a "natural fact" or condition. In contrast, the uterus transplant surgery technology being developed is based on the conviction that there is a demand for this kind of therapy in cases where women are, for instance, born without ovaries or uterus. This research work may open up for a large-scale market but there is not yet any evidence of successful pregnancies or babies born on the basis of these therapies. However, if proven to be successful, it is not unlikely that uterus transplant surgery will constitute a small niche in the ART market.

An additional concept related to uterus transplant surgery is to develop what is called tissue engineering technologies (Sharp, 2011; Hogle, 2009) to increase the supply of uterus donors. While the cases of uterus transplant surgery used living donors, the first cases of such surgery used donors from cadavers. Historically speaking there are always risks involved in using organs from cadavers that is not an issue in the case of living donors. If a uterus from a cadaver could be procured successfully, it could be combined with stem cell therapies, visionaries predict, where stem cells collected from the recipient of the uterus could be used to regenerate new tissue. In this case, the uterus serves as a scaffold onto which new stem cells are cultivated, reducing the organ rejections risks when the immunology of the uterus and the body are brought into harmony. In the wake of interest for stem cell therapies (discussed below), there are new possibilities for what Sharp (2011: 7) speaks of as "body tinkering," the use of "cells, synthetic materials, and biological factors to make functional substitutes for tissue" (Hogle, 2009: 720) in order to not only improve but to restore biological functions. Whether such concepts would be tolerable in the future – a woman re-using a dead woman's womb to give birth to a baby – is not of necessity easily predicted, but one thing that could be learned from the history of reproductive medicine and ART, representatives of the field argue, is that the boundaries for what can both be accomplished and what is being requested have been advanced over the course of the decades of assisted reproduction.

Beyond ART: regenerative medicine and the stem cell therapy promise

One of the great unanticipated consequence or parallel developments in biomedical technoscience is the advancement of stem cell therapies and the idea of regenerative medicine (Rubin, 2008; Martin, Brown, and Kraft, 2008). As discussed above, reproductive medicine is the outcome of a series of streams of research converging into the pursuit to actively promote and assist human reproduction. Little did the pioneers of assisted reproductive technologies in the 1960s and 1970s know that they would pave the way for the routines that would eventually supply embryonic stem cell researchers with the gametes needed to conduct stem cell research. Stem cell research is today one of the fields of biomedicine surrounded by the highest levels of hope and expectations, rooted in the capacity to make so-called pluripotent stem cells regenerate into various specialized cells including e.g., liver cells, heart cells, or cerebral cells. Waldby (2002) accounts for the role of stem cells in regenerative medicine:

> Stem cells are ... new biological actors, recently taking their place along genes as potent icons of promised control over biology and health. The term 'stem cell' refers to any cell that can renew tissue in the body.
>
> (Waldby, 2002: 306)

Stem cell research has been controversial as it consumes embryos and oocytes, and the presidency of George W. Bush, by and large characterized by its renewal of the Reagan era neoconservatism, was a period where American stem cell researchers had to see their jurisdictional discretion reduced on the basis of religious beliefs and ethical concerns. What Oberman, Wolf, and Zettler (2010: 261) refer to as "the politics of abortion" in the U.S., with Christian neoconservatives and pro-life activists critical of abortion rights being vastly more influential than during previous periods, stem cell research became associated with controversies regarding women's rights and legislation (Salter and Salter, 2007). The reporting of science frauds such as the case of South Korean scientists Hwang Woo Suk, consuming more than 2,000 eggs retrieved from 129 women in his embryonic stem cell research work, did not help advocates of stem cell research (Elster, 2010: 227).

While reproductive medicine and ART is clearly separated from regenerative medicine and stem cell research, there are still close connections between the two biomedical fields (Franklin, 2014, 2005; Ikemoto, 2009). For instance, as Ikemoto (2010: 238) rightly remarks, "the fertility industry created the practice that routinized human egg procurement." It is therefore little wonder that e.g., India having the least strict legislation regarding assisted reproductive technologies has become a center of stem cell research (Baradwaj and Glasner, 2009). Couples that store embryos in freezers in Sweden and that have successfully undergone the therapy and have become parents are today asked if they want to donate the embryos to embryonic stem cell research after the five-year period of storage permitted by Swedish law ends. Since these embryos are, biologically speaking, the siblings of the child already being fertilized in the laboratory and thereafter born, these decisions are not always entirely pleasant to make, but according to Swedish law, there needs to be an informed consent from the parents as the embryos cannot be stored longer than five years. This locates the couples in a "double bind" position where they have to decide whether the embryos should be transferred to the uterus, donated to scientific research, or destroyed.

One additional connection between ART and stem cell research is the presence of so-called stem cell banking services offered today in North America and Europe, where parents would store the umbilical cord blood of their new-born babies, containing stem cells, to be able to take advantage of forthcoming scientific breakthroughs in the biomedical technosciences. The scholarly literature is skeptical to say the least, thinking of these paid-for-services as the wedding of enterprising market culture and biomedical research work, leading to parents being concerned about the future health of their children to pay for what is at best a promise to be able to take advantage of what may become effective therapies in the future (Fannin, 2013; Hoeyer et al., 2009; Brown and Kraft, 2006; Glasner, 2005). In this view, an unregulated market for stem cell banking may exploit people's care for their family in terms of not really offering anything but a not negligible annual fee for the freezing of the biological materials. Again, a sociology of expectations perspective may inform how parents rationally calculate the costs and benefits of banking e.g., umbilical cord blood. From a more distant view, the costs are most likely to be higher than the benefits, and therefore biobanking may be more strictly regulated in the future (see e.g. Faulkner, 2012).

Summary and conclusion

The last two decades of advancement of experimental biomedicine is one of the most remarkable accomplishments of science and mankind as such. Today, there are spectacular things that can be accomplished on the basis of modern medicine and surgery, and contemporary humans are lucky to take advantage of a great number of therapies and medical procedures that help them live longer and happier lives. Not until the last 50 years, the issue of human infertility and sub-fertility has been grappled with on the basis of the new research findings in cytology, endocrinology, and genomics, and the early attempt to develop effective therapies was met with skepticism, based on the predominant belief in the issue of overpopulation in the post-World War II period. Today, much of this skepticism has been overcome and roughly 50 percent of couples seeking assistance can become parents.

Still, the IVF therapy also creates possibilities for e.g., gestational surrogacy which in turn surfaces a series of social issues and beliefs, most of them only in part medical but frequently grounded in institutionalized norms and inherited beliefs. Such issues include the question of whether the access to female reproductive capacities can become subject to legal contracting and monetary compensation or whether e.g., gay couples or even single men have the right to contract for such services abroad despite national legislation? These are, needless to say, not issues that are easily digested for legislative and regulatory bodies and neither are they for the wider public, at times firmly rooted in traditional norms regarding parenting and family life. At the same time, reproductive medicine and ART here follows a general biomedical trajectory wherein new medical possibilities always of necessity create their own new ethical issues and concerns, not least the trade-offs between how financial resources should be committed to various health care objectives. ART and reproductive medicine are therefore what is complicated to manage and organize as they will always create new possibilities that in turn demand further policies and regulatory practices.

Part II
Empirical studies

4   The methodology of the study

Introduction

Most research on ART is based on a social theory framework not primarily concerned with economic and managerial issues. This study seeks to understand the historical development of the clinical therapies and the various practical and ethical issues these therapies give rise to and to examine how they were handled by relevant actors. In addition, the study examines how clinicians, managers, entrepreneurs, and decision-makers actively inform and structure the field of assisted reproduction, making it what it has become today – an advanced form of biomedical treatment capable of helping around 50 percent of the involuntary childless couples and single women become parents, and an industry with a significant economic turnover. In other words, the study is not only concerned with the medical and technological aspects of the treatment or the social, cultural, and ethical consequences of these novel possibilities, but also wants to examine how actors in the industry contribute to the maintenance and development of the therapies and the service offerings to the clients. As there are few previous studies having the ambition to include these economic and financial aspects within one single study, this chapter presents the design of the study. The data collection and data analysis conducted in the day-to-day research work will be addressed in some detail.

This methodology chapter is structured into three basic sections. First, the design of the study will be accounted for, including a discussion about the concept of *field* being used extensively in sociological theory and in organization and management studies. Second, the data collection conducted is accounted for and we examine how previous studies have contributed to the way that we have collected our empirical data. Third and finally, we present the data analysis methods used as an integral part of the research work.

Design of the study

The concept of field

The greatly influential French sociologist Pierre Bourdieu is widely renowned for his use of the concept of field (French, *Champ*) as being an important element of his so-called *theory of practice*. In Bourdieu's sophisticated analytical framework, the field is the domain wherein actors are actively competing over resources and positions, using their own skills and competencies to entrench what they regard as favorable positions. Bourdieu's sociological framework is thus based on a conflictual and power-laded view of society and social domains, characterized by political struggles, the use of power, and the entrenchment of resources – material, symbolic, and financial. "The field of forces is ... a field of struggles, a socially constructed field of action in which agents equipped with different resources confront each other in order to gain access to exchange and to preserve or transform the currently prevailing relations of force," Bourdieu (2005: 199) writes. The actor operating within a particular field develops what Bourdieu speaks of as a *habitus*, the totality of endowed and learned skills and competencies that enable what Bourdieu (ibid.: 213) refers to as "a highly economical principle of action"; the habitus enables "enormous saving in calculation" as the actor can act in accordance with these learned schemes of practical action.

The habitus of the individual is also accompanied by access to what Bourdieu speaks of as *capital*, commonly discussed in terms of e.g., economic capital, symbolic capital, cultural capital, etc., i.e., various resources and competencies that can be mobilized within the field. In Bourdieu's view, certain forms of capital (e.g., reputation) are closely bound up with a specific field (e.g., cardiac surgery, snowboard riding, modern choreography) and the capital is thus situated and contextual, not easily moved between different fields. Bourdieu explains this idea in a passage not devoid of theoretical intricacies:

> *A capital does not exist and function except in relation to a field.* It confers a power over the field, over the materialized or embodied instruments of production or reproduction whose distribution constitutes the very structure of the field, and over the regularities and the rules which define the ordinary functioning of the field, and thereby over the profits engendered in it.
>
> (Bourdieu and Wacquant, 1992: 101)

The action of the agent in a particular field is therefore rooted in the habitus and represents a skilled and "intelligent" response to what Bourdieu (2005: 212) speaks of as "an actively selected aspect of the real." Reality is never given in its full scope to the individual actor, but instead the actor perceives the field from his or her horizon of meaning and takes action in order to accomplish desirable goals within this understanding. Bourdieu's analytical framework is highly influential and also seeks to reconcile the agency-structure problem present in virtually all social theory, making structural elements constitutive of the habitus that guide and organize everyday action.

What is of particular interest in this setting is the concept of the field as being the framework within which proper action is taken. There are a number of studies that draw on Bourdieu's analytical framework. Lenoir (1997: 15) uses the concept of a *scientific field* to examine the work of scientists:

The scientific field is a field of positions occupied by agents with different stances towards one another. Each field, whether politics, economics, art, literature, or science, has its own logic. To play for stakes in the scientific field requires a specific form of capital, such as educational experience and appropriate material resources.

Similarly, Ferguson's (2004) study of the prominence of French cuisine and gastronomy draws on Bourdieu's work, making a distinction between the *restaurant world*, a *culinary culture*, and the *gastronomic field* as separated, yet co-produced organizational levels capable of being studied individually:

> A *restaurant world* focuses on production of a more or less well-defined culinary product and coheres throughout networks of individuals. By contrast, a culinary culture is fixed in consumption practices and values. Finally, the gastronomic field is structured by a textual discourse that continually renegotiates the systemic tensions between production and consumption.
>
> (Ferguson, 2004: 108)

In organization and management studies, there are a number of concepts rooted in the idea of a particular "field" being the principal structuring mechanism for the agent's activities. First, *organizational fields* refer to the "immediate environments of organizations" (Edelman, Fuller, and Mara-Drita, 2001: 1595), the milieu wherein managers and co-workers create their own horizons of meaning and enact (Daft and Weick, 1984) their own social realities that they pay attention to and that guide their actions (Ansari and Phillips, 2011; DiMaggio and Powell, 1983). Second, moving to a somewhat more narrow domain, some scholars speak about *institutional fields* as a subset of the organizational field including all the instituted practices, norms and beliefs that serve to structure everyday life in organizations (Purdy and Grey, 2009; Greenwood, Suddaby, and Hinings, 2002). Third, Leblebici et al. (1991) use the term *interorganizational fields* to underline that organizational action today to a larger extent occurs in the intersection of organizations and across organizational boundaries. For instance, much innovation work is today conducted in collaborative settings, including research centers, joint ventures, and alliances, indicating that the organization is no longer enclosed and confined but must be understood as what is open towards external influences and exchanges. Changing the perspective from the organization per se to the people that populate organizations, the concept of *professional fields* denotes how certain specialized professional communities, holding licenses and legitimate jurisdictional claims, are capable of influencing how organizations structure and manage their work (Lawrence, 2004; Kitchener, 2002). By and large, there is a perceived difficult relationship between professional communities and managerial initiatives and numerous studies reveal ongoing jurisdictional struggles between professionals (e.g., physicians in health care organizations and hospital directors).

More recently, sociologists such as Neil Fligstein and Doug McAdam have proposed what they refer to as a *field theory* as a fruitful analytical framework for studies of organizations. While Bourdieu's theory of practice strongly stresses conflicts and struggles within specific fields, Fligstein and McAdam (2012) would not assume that is always of necessity the case, but the role and influence of conflicts is per se an empirical question. The study of the Swedish reproductive medicine and ART field demonstrates that there is more evidence of consensus and collaboration between both professionals and regulatory bodies and agencies and across the private–public domain than there is conflict and controversies. Such findings do not indicate that there are no sources of discussions or debates, but by and large there are other social fields that are possibly characterized by higher degrees of conflict (e.g., politics, the media market, the finance market). Given these results, accounted for in Part II of this volume, we recognize the contributions of Pierre Bourdieu to the understanding of the field as the domain wherein social and professional action takes place and is recognized, but we still believe the "theory of fields," as advocated by Fligstein and McAdam (2012), is more helpful in capturing the variety of the empirical data.

The Swedish reproductive medicine and assisted reproduction field includes a variety of firms, professional communities, regulatory agencies, political bodies such as parties and the parliament, activist groups, patient groups, and what actor-network theorists speak of as *quasi-objects* (a term introduced by philosopher Michel Serres, 1982: 225) and *actants*, objects including, in this case, biomedical entities such as sperm, eggs, and embryos that in themselves lack the capacity of agency but nevertheless are being introduced as relevant social and biomedical actors. In other words, this field includes not only firms and professional communities but instead there is a wide variety of actors that preferably should be properly integrated within one single analytical framework. We believe the concept of field and field theory provides such analytical possibilities, and we therefore follow Heilbron, Verheul and Quak (2013) and Driessens (2013) who advocate and use field theory in their empirical research work.

Data collection

Design of the study. The present study is based on a case study methodology (David, 2006; Stake, 1996). The principal data collection methods were interviews with actors working in the field in either assisted reproduction clinics or in academic reproductive medicine departments. Interviewing (Holstein and Gubrium, 2003; Kvale, 1996) has been used previously in studies of in vitro fertilization practices (Becker, 2000; Cussins, 1996, 1998), of egg donation agencies and sperm banks (Almeling, 2011; Snowdon, 1994), and studies of surrogacy services (Pande, 2009, 2010). In total, there are six public clinics and ten private clinics in the whole of Sweden employing 150–200 persons *in toto*. For this reason we chose interviewees from a range of different clinics, in order to gain knowledge of as much of the national field as possible. The number of interviewees from each clinic varied from one to seven.

One of the trickiest parts for the practicing researcher is to get a firm hold of what is happening in the field, to get a glimpse of what actually occurs rather than being provided with formal statements regarding the activities. This practical research concern is grounded in an epistemological problem that has several layers that need to be addressed. First of all, there is the *practical problem* of getting access to either interview data or observational data, that is, to be able to claim some of the time from normally quite busy practitioners otherwise having relatively limited interests in contributing to scholarly research. This challenge commonly translates into a time-consuming and in many ways stressful procedure where emails are sent and telephone calls are made, but in most cases this is manageable with a little bit of *sang froid* and persistency. A more cumbersome *epistemological problem* is addressed by Howard Becker (1996): how we can listen to what people say and observe what they do without inscribing any preconceived ideas or prejudice into what they are trying to accomplish. We can here cite Becker at length:

> [W]e *always* describe how they [people studied] interpret the events they participate in, so the only question is not whether we should, but how accurately we do it. We can find out, not with perfect accuracy, but better than zero, what people think they are doing, what meanings they give to the objects and events and people in their lives and experience. We do that by talking to them, in formal and informal interviews, in quick exchanges while we participate and observe their ordinary activities, and by watching and listening as they go about their business; we can even do it by giving them questionnaires which let them say what their meanings are or choose between meanings we give them as possibilities. To anticipate a later point, the nearer we get to the conditions in which they actually do attribute meanings to objects and events, the more accurate our descriptions of those meanings are likely to be.
>
> (Becker, 1996: 58)

For Becker (1996), researchers are always at risk of projecting their preconceived ideas onto the informants, but the closer the researcher is to the practitioners, the easier it is to gain a comprehensive understanding of their life world and their beliefs and choices. At the same time as a certain proximity is commonly recommended in the research methodology, this closeness is by no means of necessity leading to the privileged access to spectacular events that would not otherwise be revealed to outsiders. On the contrary, as Van Maanen (1979: 543) argues, despite the best intentions of the researcher, fieldwork "almost always boils down to series of endless conversations intersected by a few major events and a host of less formidable ones."

This perceived lack of spectacular findings, the demon of all ethnographers and empirical researchers enduring a sense of wasting their best years sitting in organizations to observe what is conspicuously insignificant, actually comes in two versions. First, John Law (1994: 43–44) speaks of "the ethnographer's anxiety" to denote this sense of not being able to acquire any particularly interesting research findings and that everything of notoriety is taking place elsewhere; "Where the ethnographer is, the Action is not," Law (1994: 45) says.

On the other hand, as Karin Knorr Cetina (1983: 123) has made clear, in many cases the ethnographer encounters not precisely "a set of parameters which neatly specify [the work] process," but in many cases the laboratory work is messy, disorderly, and complicated to understand, and only after spending several months in the laboratory can the researcher learn that much of the professional work of the scientist is "concerned with counteracting and remedying this disorder." While the world encountered by Law's (1994) researcher is inert and dull, the laboratory of Knorr Cetina is overwhelmingly complicated to cognitively process and fully understand in all details.

The research literature genre of ethnography is defined by Watson (2011: 205. Emphasis in the original) accordingly: "[A] *style of social science writing which draws upon the writer's close observation of and involvement with people in a particular social setting and relates the words spoken and the practices observed or experienced to the overall cultural framework within which they occurred.*" This definition underlines the "writer's role" in reporting what he or she believes are worthy of being noted, and the very genre of ethnography is closely bound up with the idea of what Foucault (1973) – addressing the epistemology of medical diagnoses – refers to as "a speaking eye." Says Van Maanen (2011: 222):

> Ethnography's focus on the 'empirical' alongside its 'I-witnessing' – meaning its intense reliance on personalized seeing, hearing, and experiencing in specific social settings – has always generated something of a hostility to generalizations and abstractions not connected to immersion in situated detail.

This "reporting" (Watson, 2011) and "witnessing" (Van Maanen, 2011) unfolds quite differently in the two cases of Law (1994) and Knorr Cetina (1983). In the former case, theories are likely to inform the ethnographer's possibly more desperate search for significant events and occurrences, while in the latter case the ethnographer is fully equipped with understanding what is "going on" in the laboratory. In the former case, when theories become the last resort for the researcher to justify further empirical research work, in the latter case a principal difficulty is that much professional work, not least in scientific communities, demands expertise and qualifications that the researcher cannot be expected to fully acquire within the stipulated time. As the science and technology studies literature has accounted for time and again, professional research skills are acquired slowly and only through practice and in many cases, it remains inarticulate as such skills are residing in ways of doing and looking (e.g., Myers, 2008; Roth, 2005; Jordan and Lynch, 1992).

Despite all these worries and caveats regarding the possibilities for acquiring an understanding for what happens in the field, in organizations and in professional communities, research work can still provide some useful insight into a world of practice. It is meaningful to question claims regarding objectivity and truth in research communities, but to endorse the idea of the researcher gains no insights whatsoever and seems overly unproductive and counterintuitive. This pragmatist epistemology based on a skeptical attitude towards final or unconditional truth-claims (see e.g., Rorty, 1989) also characterizes the uses of the interview materials reported in the empirical part of this volume. Atkinson and Coffrey (2003: 110) suggest that researchers should not assume that "what is done should enjoy primacy over what is said," i.e., that there is a qualitative ranking of observations and interview materials. Instead, Atkinson and Coffrey (2003) propose that "actions" are understandable because "they can be talked about." In other words, observations of activities and the talk about them are complementary inasmuch as they serve to bridge the domains of materiality and embodiment and human cognitions and narrative practices – the storytelling that pertains to all actual work. At the same time, Atkinson and Coffrey (2003: 117) continue, "[w]e cannot take the interview as a proxy for action." As there is always a certain deviation between espoused theories and theories-in-use (Argyris and Schön, 1978), interviews serve the role of being the occasion in which the informants "[c]onstruct themselves and others as particular forms of moral agents" (Atkinson and Coffrey, 2003: 116).

A common sense understanding of the deviations between what is said and what is done as what is untruthful, immoral, or an evidence of mere hypocrisy, but a pragmatist epistemology and a behavioral model of human action is less eager to denounce such events as being morally questionable as human beings are always thrown into the process wherein actions and meaning construction are co-produced while rarely being fully synchronized; action and meaning are thus related but not tightly bounded. As a consequence, Suddaby (2006: 635) writes, interviews are "[a] means of eliciting information on the social situation under examination." This loose coupling between action and meaning opens up for what Suddaby (2006: 636) refers to as an "interpretativist ontology," wherein human beings do not "passively react to an external reality" but instead they do their best to "[i]mpose their internal perceptions and ideals of the external world and, in so doing, actively create their realities." In other words, interviews are not really accounting for objectively true facts, nor are they based on mere fantasies or figments of the imagination of the interviewees, but what oscillates between these end-points on the continuum in the pursuit to create meaning both for themselves and the interviewer they encounter. The absolute majority of cases want to inform and help the best they can.

The use of documents

As has been demonstrated by historians of media (Goody, 1986; Ong, 1982; Innes, 1972) and organization researchers (Yates, 1989), the advance of writing and the production of textual documents and archives precedes the growth of more differentiated human societies and larger and more sophisticated organization forms. More recently, scholars in the field of management communication (e.g., Ashcraft, Kuhn, and Cooren, 2009) have emphasized the role of written documents and what Cooren (2004) has referred to as *textual agency* for the structuring of organizations. Cooren (2004: 375) argues that organizational activities are "discursively structured" and therefore all forms of written texts including formal documents (e.g., contracts), memos, checklists, and instructions can "display forms of agency." What Cooren speaks of as a "textual agency approach" in organizations studies constitutes an organization as "a hybrid of human and nonhuman contributions." Created by human beings, various texts "[p]articipate in the channeling of behaviors, constitute and stabilize organizational pathways, and broadcast information/orders," Cooren (2004: 388) proposes. In addition, these textual documents "enable delegation" through what Cooren calls "tele-action" and "tele-communication," action and communication "from afar," at a distance from the actual practices. Carruthers and Espeland (1991: 56) suggest that what is presented in a written form appear to be more "fixed" than what is presented orally, and consequently, the interpretation of written documents typically presumes that the meaning of the text is more static and less dependent on specific audiences than in the oral statement. Written documents are thus one tool for structuring and determining e.g., organizational practices as they are prescribed in manuals and other forms of instructive documents.

Faulkner (2012) proposes that documents contain performative capacities as e.g., legislative texts and documents are the outcome from sociopolitical and technoscientific debates and negotiations. These documents are thus both the endpoint of such political discussions and the blueprint for the activities that are supposed to follow the determination of the political decisions and recommendation. "Legislative documents can be understood as working performatively. They cannot be understood as simply the repository of sets of textual prohibitive and enabling law – their performativity is much richer than this," Faulkner (2012: 755) says. Legal scholars such as Edelman (1990, 1992) similarly stress how legal texts are capable of producing social effects that may be both wider and different from what the legislators initially wanted to accomplish, making legal texts somewhat imprecise tools for shaping social action. Faulkner (2012: 755) makes a distinction between *texts*, which are open to e.g., discourse or textual analyses and documents, and *documents*, which "play an active part as a vehicle of a given political system."

Previous studies show that various forms of documents do play a key role in structuring everyday work in organizations. Barley and Bechky's (1994) study of laboratory technicians relied extensively on forms of documentation as a "backbone technology" to keep the laboratory functional and operative, keeping the multiple sources of errors and failure that threatened the production of scientific data at bay. Nicolini, Mengis, and Swan's (2012: 625) study of the role of material objects in cross-disciplinary collaborations in knowledge-intensive work suggests that documents serve the role of what they refer to as "tertiary objects of collaboration," being part of the infrastructure that supports collaborate work.

In the present study of ART, there are a great number of legal and regulatory bodies, ethical councils, and professional organizations that issue reports and recommendations regarding everyday practices and forthcoming scientific possibilities, and there are a great number of documents that can be examined. We have not been able to exhaust this source of empirical material but have rather used a few documents that we have acquired as part of the interview work. First, we have been given accounting data from one of the major companies in the industry to be able to examine the costs structure of the operations. Such internal memos have provided us with a first-hand account of how private companies in the industry need to carefully monitor their costs and ensure that there is a sufficient amount of treatment cycles conducted annually to cover all the costs and to generate a profit. Second, we have made use of a report issued by the State of Sweden's Medical Ethical Council (SSMEC) and commissioned by the Ministry of Health and Social Affairs. This report presents the council's recommendations regarding the legal frameworks regulating the industry, including the various reservations made by medical experts and political representatives. Access to this document provides an immediate insight into the medical–ethical discussions and considerations made, including the framing of particular ethical problems among the council's members. Taken together, these documents make important contributions to the overall understanding of the industry being subject to analysis.

Practical data collection

The data include 47 interviewees in nine different ART clinics in Sweden, public as well as private, as well as researchers in the field of reproductive medicine, politicians, government officials, interest group representatives, company representatives and patients. Interviews were structured by an interview guide, composed of both questions derived from the literature on assisted reproduction and wider theoretical interest pertaining to the organization of the clinics. All interviews were conducted in situ, tape-recorded, and lasted around one hour, with some interviews lasting for as long as one and a half hours. Table 4.1 summarizes information on the types of interviewees included in the study.

Table 4.1 Interviewees participating in the study

	Public	Private	
Physicians/gynecologists, with or without PhD	5	8	
Laboratory employees, with or without PhD	8	2	
Midwives, information specialist	1	1	
Psychologist	1		
Administrators	1	2	
Policy-maker, regulatory body	6		
Companies delivering technology and drugs for ART		2	
Patients' interest groups	4	NA	
Patients	NA	6	
Number of interviewees per category/in total	**26**	**21**	**47**

Practical data analysis

Interviews were transcribed by a professional transcriber and were coded individually by two senior researchers. The interview excerpts were first coded (Strauss and Corbin, 1998) on the basis of the basic content of the quote and as all transcripts were divided in such encoded passages, they were structured into larger "second-order" categories serving to interrelate the theoretical framework and the empirical material (see e.g., Heyl, 2001; Spradley, 1979, Chapter 8). Examples of such codes were "technological developments," "policy and regulations," and "scientific practices." These second-order categories were used to "emplot" (White, 1987) the data into a narrative about how legal and regulatory changes are influencing the organization of assisted reproduction clinics.

5   Creating institutions
Advocating and promoting new ART

Introduction

In the first of the three empirical chapters, the concept of institutional work aimed at creating novel institutions and practices will be addressed. As explained at the end of Chapter 2 in Part I of the book, institutional creation is the process wherein primarily insiders, i.e., professionals and experts, engage in the development and advancement of new clinical practices, technologies, and processes that serve to open up for new clinical possibilities and new market segments. In this chapter, three forms of institutional creation will be examined. The first case addresses how a relatively mature technology, the freezing of ova, in itself relatively uncontroversial today as the technology has proved its efficacy and safety over the decades, has become used for a new purpose. The new purpose is to encourage younger women, preferably below the age of 30, to retrieve eggs from their ovaries and to store them in the laboratory as a form of insurance against future infertility problems. This procedure is referred to as a *social freezing* in the field.

The second case addresses the proposed extended use of a technology already in use, pre-implantation genetic diagnostics/screening (PGD/PGS), the procedure to examine the genome of the embryo prior to the selection and transfer of one embryo to the womb. In this case, the very idea of using PGD/PGS is controversial as some policy-makers and others tend to associate the technique with what at times is referred to as eugenic medicine associated with an unwarranted expansion of how medical technologies are used to shape and inform human life, arguably in ways that violate norms about human dignity. Against the history of eugenic medicine, PGD/PGS, while it may be helpful to increase precision of the therapy when being used wisely and under controlled conditions, the technology remains controversial on the basis of its associations.

Third and finally, the far more innovative and even spectacular wedding of organ transplant surgery and reproductive medicine in the uterus transplantation project located at the Sahlgrenska University Hospital in Gothenburg, Sweden, will be addressed. The uterus transplantation project aims to transfer a uterus from one donor to a recipient with the intention of making the recipient become a mother by giving birth to a baby. This project holds the promise of helping women born without a functioning uterus or suffering from injuries and generally speaking extends the horizon for reproductive medicine and ART. The sheer scope of this project unsurprisingly leads to many worried comments and objections and there is ample room for all sorts of debates on the basis of the idea of where the line of demarcation between what are justifiable and too far-driven biomedical activities when it comes to the creation of human life should be drawn. Regardless of such criticism, always accompanying institutional work aimed at creating new possibilities, the uterus transplantation project remains one of the most intriguing projects in the field for the time being, receiving attention from the international press.

Case 1: Social freezing – balancing ethical concerns and reproductive and commercial possibilities when storing human eggs

Common sense thinking and ethical concerns

IVF has today been successfully used as a clinical practice for more than three and a half decades and hundreds of thousands of children fertilized in the laboratory are born annually. If the costs for IVF therapies had been lower and available for a larger proportion of the global human population, the demographic and clinical consequences of IVF would be even more salient. Representatives of the clinics and regulatory bodies widely claim that today, IVF as a clinical practice is no longer controversial and all the initial concerns regarding "test-tube babies" and "baby factories" have waned as the clinical practices have demonstrated its efficacy and safety. At the same time as reproductive medicine and IVF therapies have been widely recognized, the field of reproductive medicine is still at times treated as representing what one of the interviewees referred to as "luxury health care":

> We offer 'luxury health care.' I have had these incredibly animated discussions with my best friend who is a diabetes physician. She believes what I do to be luxury. It is 'no human right to have children' … But that represents an economic view, and that is in most cases prioritized above everything else.
>
> (Resident Surgery and Gynecology,
> Medical director, IVF Sweden)

A professor in reproductive medicine, shared this experience: "Many people believe that reproductive medicine handles luxury problems" (Professor #2, reproductive medicine). Reproductive medicine treats patients that are not by definition ill but rather share the medical condition of suffering from sub-fertility, and in comparison to e.g., the field of cancer medicine and therapy, the predicament of childlessness is, in this lay account, less problematic. The professor argued that it was easy for an outsider, in particular when having children of their own, to underrate the psychological and social costs of not being able to become parents: "We meet these patients, while a middle aged man, say an internal medicine physician with four children of his own, may not think this is relevant. 'Why don't these poor women just adopt instead?'" (Professor #2, reproductive medicine). In addition, no matter whether IVF is a "luxury therapy" or not, there are studies demonstrating the economic rationale in offering IVF treatment:

> It has been clearly proven that every IVF child has covered its own health care costs within a year, more or less. You produce a new [future] taxpayer. Unless the parents could have their child, they would have suffered from psychological disorders to a higher extent. That in turn would have affected the labour market in terms of sick leave and that.
>
> (Resident Surgery and Gynecology,
> Medical director, Private IVF company)

One of the direct consequences of the marginalization of reproductive medicine was the difficulties involved in raising research funds, a long-standing concern in the field:

> The concern is, both in Sweden and abroad, that there is not enough funding. If you work in the field of reproductive medicine, you have a hard time getting research grants. The easiest field is in cardiovascular research and in cancer … Bob Edwards' [Nobel Prize laureate and pioneer in reproductive medicine] story was that he had a real hard time trying … [the Medical Research Council members said] 'Why can't you just continue to work on these contraception pills?'
>
> (Professor #2, reproductive medicine)

In addition to common sense thinking, stating that "there are already so many children in this world, and why can't these people just adopt?", the field of reproductive medicine and its clinical branch, also have to respond to the various ethical and medical issues addressed by the regulatory bodies that monitor the clinics. Interviews with a member of the State of Sweden's Bioethical Advisory Board, an advisory body that examined ethical issues pertaining to reproductive medicine to prepare legislating bodies for their decisions, revealed that ideas regarding what is "natural" and what is not were articulated in the discussions also in these expert communities:

> These discussions cannot be summarized in a few sentences, but you may say that the concepts of what is 'natural' and what is 'unnatural' plays a role. IVF as a method has been accepted as a clinical method ... [But] that is an 'unnatural' method ... so it is a matter of being on a slippery slope. In all ethical discussions, there are slippery slopes ... If you change the ethical norms, the 'slippery slope argument' is always articulated. What will happen in the next stage? A majority of the council made this argument regarding altruistic surrogacy.
>
> (Director #1, State of Sweden
> Bioethical Advisory Board)

"Slippery slope arguments" are always part of ethical debates structured around the question "if we tolerate this practice, what would be the implications in the next phase?," and in e.g., the case of so-called altruistic gestational surrogacy being one recent issue of discussion, there was, for instance, a concern that surrogacy on a voluntary basis would legitimize *all kinds* of surrogacy services, leading to a potential upsurge in demand also for commercial surrogacy.

The concept of nature and its allegedly primordial qualities would be a qualified starting point for biomedical and bioethical discussions. However, it is at the same time a somewhat misplaced concept as technoscience at large and advanced biomedicine has little to do with a common sense view of nature, but always already seeks to intervene and manipulate the human biological organism. In reproductive medicine, there are also social and cultural norms and religious beliefs that interfere with the analysis, leading to animated ethical discussions. In order to avoid a moralist stance regarding, for instance, who should be eligible for IVF therapies (in Sweden, lesbian couples were not legally permitted to undergo IVF therapies until 2006, and single women were excluded until July 2015), the discussion centers on the safety and interests of the unborn child:

> Our discussions start very much in a concern for safety. What do we know about the effects? ... For example, what do we know

about providing IVF to 40–45 year old persons. Is there an increased risk for the mother and the child, and in such cases you need to return to the scientific literature to check. In the case of uterus transplantation, we had to do this review of the scientific literature.

(Board member #1, State of Sweden
Bioethical Advisory Board)

The Bioethical Advisory Board member thought the practitioners in the field of reproductive medicine tended to underrate the risks in their enthusiastic accounts of research-in-progress and the new possibilities being developed. As a consequence, the Bioethical Advisory Board had to take on the responsibility to actively examine both the research practices and its clinical application from all conceivable perspectives:

We believe the researchers … tend to exaggerate and emphasize the positive effects, whereas safety issues are not handled accordingly … [For example] we organized a workshop on neuroethics and it is amazing what things they may accomplish with these implanted electrodes, but it is reasonable to assume that it also entails a few risks. There was not very much said about those risks during the day.

(Director #1, State of Sweden
Bioethical Advisory Board)

This praise of what is in the making is an irreducible element of all scientific pursuit, but it is perhaps also indicative of the need to create new and interesting research concepts and therapeutic practices that attract new talent to mature or even stagnating scientific fields. The professor in reproductive medicine addressed this concern:

It is complicated to recruit young physicians to the IVF field today. When [the pioneers of IVF] started all this, this was what everybody wanted to do because there were so many exciting things, but now … not much happens in reproductive medicine … Nothing spectacular, anyway.

(Professor #2, reproductive medicine)

The interviewed regulatory bodies understood this dynamic of biomedical fields and disciplines but still served the role of moderating the more visionary projects in order to counteract the general public's concern regarding the degrees of freedom when intervening into human biological organisms. No domain of biomedical research can be sheltered from this regulatory control, the Bioethical Advisory Board director made clear: "There are many visionaries who want to spend time talking about the future and future methods and engineered gametes and all that. But there needs to be some limitations, damn it!" (Director #1, State of Sweden Bioethical Advisory Board).

The promise and predicament of social freezing

One method or clinical service that would add value to the IVF clinics and enhance their performance but that was yet surrounded by many ethical and regulatory concerns was the process of *social freezing*. Practically speaking, social freezing is a traditional IVF therapy being temporarily postponed for a number of years in between the egg retrieval and the fertilization and embryo growth. In that respect, social freezing relies on a well-established standard procedure, not itself being particularly complicated. It is only quite recently that the methods to freeze unfertilized eggs have been developed, offering the possibility of a "postponed pregnancy." The concern is that this new reproductive medical service demands younger women to actively anticipate and handle their own reproductive futures and to make an investment decision regarding their own possibilities of future motherhood.

In addition to this possibility – or even norm – regarding an enterprising attitude towards one's reproductive future, the very retrieval of the eggs demand first a hormone therapy that stimulates the ovulation (Cussins, 1998) – at times, in unfortunate situations, leading to Ovarian Hyperstimulation Syndrome (OHSS), that can demand hospitalization, especially for Asian women (Oberman, Wolf, and Zettler, 2010: 253) – and the process where the eggs are collected from the ovaries, widely regarded as an unpleasant and painful experience. Also, because the freezing methods are relatively new, the effectiveness of this storage may not be fully guaranteed. The question then remains whether IVF clinics and regulatory bodies should encourage younger women to engage with social freezing to secure their future chances of becoming parents?

First of all, the Swedish legislation was both ambiguous and included limitations. As one gynecologist argued, the Swedish legislation which maximizes freezing time for gametes and embryos to five years deviated from the legislation of other countries: "This regulatory framework [regarding freezing] is very limiting ... Why on earth is this done still when the countries around us have increased to ten years? In Finland it's ten years; in the UK, ten years." Practically speaking, if a woman retrieves eggs at the age of 29, a quite reasonable age for making such a decision, the interviewees argued, then she would have to make use of her eggs by 34. But many couples seeking assisted reproduction are closer to 40 than 35, and many private clinics treat women older than 40. For this reason, the legislation complicates the practical use of social freezing.

In addition, one interviewee representing one of the private clinics argued that the legislation was unclear regarding social freezing: "This issue is not regulated by law ... There are many situations [where social freezing is an attractive option], from getting cancer to being offered this career position in Brussels, to where you have a relationship with a man not being interested in having children" (Resident Surgery and Gynecology, Medical director, Private Clinic). The same interviewee saw both an opportunity to help the despairing couples that visited the clinic and a business case in both providing paid-for social freezing services and the possibility to, in the future, accomplish better clinical results when ova retrieved at a younger age would have been used in the IVF therapy. He preferred to speak about social freezing as "auto-donation":

> The last year, we have been engaged in this thing being referred to as social egg freezing. We had this work group that I have been part of ... Two clinics so far offer this service [in this city]. I prefer to call it auto-donation because just like you may donate blood prior to an operation, you may also donate eggs you may need. In the best case, you would not need them.
>
> (Resident Surgery and Gynecology,
> Medical director, IVF Sweden)

Many of the interviewees encountering patients on a daily basis argued that they believed there was a surprisingly low awareness of the biological conditions for human reproduction. One of the nurses said she had countless disheartening discussions with women above the age of 40 about their limited chances of becoming mothers through giving birth, and that these women were surprised to learn about their declining reproductive capacities and how limited the IVF therapies were when making use of "older" oocytes. These interviewees called for better education regarding human reproduction and pointed at the value of campaigns reminding e.g., career women in metropolitan areas – the principal client group of IVF clinics – to pay attention to their reproductive capacities. Given these concerns and the postponement of parenthood more largely as a contemporary trend, these were opportunities for clinical services such as social freezing:

> Undoubtedly social freezing will increase. That is one thing I have considered myself. And my conclusion is, Why not? Studies show that it is socioeconomically beneficial if a twenty-five year old freezes her eggs and saves them. If she returns when she's thirty-eight, then her eggs are still young.
>
> (Gynecologist, Clinic #5)

Not everyone was equally enthusiastic about this new service. One of the gynecologists spoke of social freezing as a form of "medicalization" wherein younger women, in addition to everything else they needed to be concerned about, would be expected to plan and monitor their own reproductive futures:

> Social freezing gives me the creeps ... Should we really medicalize life to that extent? ... But there are cases I can accept but those are less 'social' than 'medical', such as in the case of people who have cancer.
>
> (Gynecologist, Founder of Clinic #7)

A professor in reproductive medicine, having two daughters herself, claimed that it would be more helpful for younger women if societal norms enabled them to become mothers below the age of 30 instead of postponing parenthood until the late 30s. The reasons for postponing motherhood was described as the effect of a career-oriented work life characterized by an inability to recognize basic human biological needs and demands. Many of the interviewees argued it was important to protect younger women from being burdened by the decision of anticipating future infertility problems, as indicated by the interview excerpt below:

> Q: May I ask at what age would be the best to procure the eggs and freeze them at a reasonable cost?
> A: Around 30

Q. Not earlier?

A: Then the woman is not yet aware she's not able to make it on time. We mustn't exploit a young woman's parents and expose her for risks. The risks are not substantial, but it is still an ethical issue. (Professor and reproductive medicine researcher, University Hospital, Sweden)

Implementing legal or public health care provision restrictions or enabling the use of new technologies such as social freezing, was discussed by our interviewees working as local politicians and administrators of regional government bodies dealing with health care. One politician expressed respect for those who are willing to go to great lengths to be able to have children. The importance of this issue stood out, and the level of engagement among the patient groups was described as higher compared to other areas of health care:

Q: Is this issue pretty similar or is it different from other health care issues?

A: No, I think it is different. It engages people so enormously. (Why do you think that is?) I think it has to do that you so desperately want to have children, it feels very important, and they describe how they have psychological and all kinds of problems. I think there is something to that. I think you have to respect that too. (Regional politician working with health care issues)

The politician went on to explain that new technologies based on research developments are meant to improve people's lives, and thus should be supported. In the case of IVF resistance was described as being based on ideas of infertility not being a serious problem, and that society should not take responsibility for guaranteeing individuals' possibility of having children. However, this politician was generally positive about new research-based technologies:

We have discussed this and of course there are always those who say 'Well, it isn't a human right to have children.' But I mean, at the same time this becomes a non-sustainable situation when you consider that we have research and development in society in order to help people with different things. I mean, all of health care is based on that we research and improve and if we then can't utilize

those medicines and technologies that emerge it feels a little ... My
hope is anyway that research will lead to improving people's lives.
(Regional politician working with health care issues)

In the public health care administration bodies, the research support for
new technologies was also emphasized. However, it was the
effectiveness of new treatments in relation to their costs that one
administrator said that they paid most attention to: "We follow the
development of research that could have an impact on our decisions,
because it is of course an issue of getting a good utility for a reasonable
cost" (Health care administrator for a regional government body). All
new technologies that improved the lives of the citizens were thus
scrutinized when it came to what was seen as reasonable to pay for the
added usefulness that they provided to potential patients, which is not
surprising in a public welfare state financed through taxes.

In summary, social freezing would on the one hand increase the
chances of women in their late 30s becoming parents if they could use
ova being retrieved at a younger age. On the other hand, there are legal,
regulatory, ethical, and financial factors to consider when deciding
whether social freezing should be promoted as a legitimate ART or not.
Moreover, there are perhaps not so much biomedical issues to address
as social freezing relies on similar standard operation procedures to that
of IVF therapies (hormone therapies, egg retrieval, the storage of the ova
in freezers) as there are ethical and social concerns. First of all, neither the
community of reproductive medicine professionals, nor politicians have
finally made up their minds regarding social freezing, but all parts, also
including bioethicists, point at both benefits, e.g., better clinical results in
future IVF therapies, and social costs, e.g., the increased pressure on
younger women and their parents/spouses to treat reproductive
capacities as what needs to be actively managed.

The representatives of private clinics, making their return on investment
on the basis of fees may be understood to be unconditional supporters of
social freezing as that would add another clinical service to their offerings,
but these clinics are already today running at a profit and foresee no
decline in demand for IVF therapies as more and more couples, especially
in the larger cities, postpone their parenthood. Instead, they tend to
regard social freezing as a vehicle for improving the chances of successful
IVF therapies in the future. As the private clinics tend to receive couples
that have already failed their treatment in the public sector clinics, have
one child, or are above the age limits enacted by the public health care

sector, private clinic representatives have good reasons beyond the short-term profit-motive to endorse clinical practices that may increase the chances of successful IVF treatment.

In other words, new biomedical and reproductive medicine concepts such as social freezing must be understood as the outcome from institutional work engaging a variety of actors which in turn make reference to and invoke various norms, beliefs, opportunities, technologies, tools, biochemical compounds and substances (e.g., media) in order to jointly determine what clinical practices are to be legitimized and promoted and what groups should be made eligible for the therapy. For instance, according to Swedish law, single women are not eligible for IVF therapy, but if social freezing was widely promoted, it would be unreasonable to expect that a woman storing her eggs be able to report what man or woman she predicts would be her partner and the other parent of the yet unborn child to be fertilized in perhaps ten years in the future. Such regulatory intricacies are always of necessity part of the institutional work that actors need to orchestrate. Reproductive medicine and other biomedical fields create new opportunities, but these new opportunities also beget their own controversies and debates.

The social and economic consequences of social freezing

As detailed by a substantial feminist literature, just like many other concepts developed within reproductive medicine, social freezing can be interpreted as being both liberating and repressive. Martin (2010: 526) refers to social freezing with the more formal, medical term "oocyte cryopreservation" and says this new method is based on the novel concept of "anticipated infertility" (ibid.: 527). The egg freezer is here "split in two," Martin (ibid.: 526) writes: "Her younger self is the egg donor, her older self the recipient, the two selves separated by time and experience." Seen in this view, Martin (ibid.: 526) argues, "egg freezing is a concise illustration of how the medicalization of women's bodies and bodily processes masks a host of cultural anxieties about ageing, illness, reproduction, and risk."

While Martin (2010) recognizes the value of social freezing in the case of women undergoing cancer treatment, the method is expanding, as in so many other cases where medicalization intervenes, to include also other groups, in this case those not even suffering from a medical condition but instead operating under particular social and cultural conditions that render pregnancies and parenting problematic. That is, this targeted group of younger women is not battling cancer but give priority to "education, career, and the search for 'Mr. Right'" (ibid.: 537):

> Once a condition is medicalized, its boundaries are not static; rather, the category itself is subject to expansion ... Technologies developed to assist one group of people with particular biomedical needs are applied to other populations with different needs and situations.
>
> (Martin, 2010: 528)

The meaning of fertility and infertility has become redefined, according to Martin.

As a consequence of this medicalization of human reproduction and the opening up of new segments in the market, a new vocabulary including terms such as "fertility preservation" – in 2009 alone, there were 299 articles published using the term, Martin (2010: 533) reports – serves as the ideological framework that naturalizes social freezing: "'Fertility preservation' is ... a misnomer," Martin (ibid.) writes. She continues:

> Women who use their own thawed eggs because they cannot conceive of their own are no more fertile than those women who use donated eggs for the same reason. What *has* been preserved is not their fertility, but the genetic connection. 'Fertility' is here redefined as not the ability to spontaneously conceive and carry a pregnancy, but the ability to transmit one's genetic material to future generations.

In Martin's (2010: 533) view, social freezing is thus primarily a commercial service that purports to benefit "healthy young women who wish to pause their biological clocks," and thereby conceals the medicalization of human reproduction through the marketing of the service as a matter of empowering women and offering them the choice to manage their own reproductive capacities through oocyte cryopresevation. "As a tool of risk management, egg freezing is a technological remedy of displacement, ameliorating fears of childlessness and the reproductive and genetic unknown at the same time it puts women's bodies and bank accounts at risk," Martin (ibid.: 540) summarizes.

In addition, Martin stresses the underlying financialized cost–benefit calculation practices that are implied in social freezing: "Financial optimization has become another category to consider in the risk of cost–benefit analysis of biomedicine. Egg freezing, similar to other forms of autologous tissue banking, is future-oriented, becoming more valuable frozen and stored than left to age contained within the body" (Martin, 2010: 540). Social freezing would enhance individual possibilities for becoming a parent, while at the same time it burdens the individual with decisions that may or may not prove to be of great importance in the future. In other words, by banking her human eggs, the individual woman can on the one hand take advantage of new biomedical possibilities, while on the other hand, she succumbs to a general tendency in the bioeconomy to store and bank biological tissues and reproductive materials to be able to anticipate future events.

In addition to reproductive material (gametes), there is today a wide variety of human tissue being stored in commercial tissue banks (Waldby and Mitchell, 2006), including the highly controversial case of umbilical cord blood containing human stem cells (Brown and Kraft, 2006: Glasner, 2005). Fannin (2013) addresses this tendency to store biological material (i.e., stem cells) as a form of "hoarding," a term used by Karl Marx to denote the capitalist who withholds capital from its circulation and stores it at safe distance from everyday economic matters. For Fanning (2013: 44) stem cell banking is "[e]xemplary of the reconceptualization of health and health care as a form of individualized risk management of future uncertainty." Individuals are no longer expected to trust their own bodies and to treat them as healthy and unproblematic but instead to actively anticipate their decline or failures through the storing of biological matter that holds the potential, the marketing materials ensure, to take advantage of future thrusts in biomedical technoscience. "If insurance promises to provide financial compensation for future unforeseen events, the stem cell banking account similarly promises an individually tailored therapy whose potential profits will be measured in the benefits of extended health," Fannin (ibid.) argues.

Social freezing is operating in accordance with a similar logic with the important difference that IVF therapies, as opposed to the field of regenerative medicine making use of stem cell therapies, are already successfully developed and clinically evaluated. At the same time, interviewees skeptical towards the social freezing service are anxious to protect younger women from "hoarding" reproductive materials and instead rearticulate the "sub-fertility problem" in terms of the failure to align human biological processes, social expectations, and lifestyles in the contemporary era. In this view, social freezing represents a form of "filter in the chimney" solution to reproductive challenges, making the use of technoscientific resources handle what are at the bottom line cultural and social issues. The costs for this maneuver are that younger women are exposed to unreasonable expectations in terms of managing and overseeing their own reproductive futures. On the other hand, when treating social freezing more strictly as a biomedical solution to a clinical problem – more mature eggs are less easily fertilized and leading to successful pregnancies than less mature eggs – social freezing is a rational and reasonable solution to identified social and individual problems and should therefore be actively handled by regulatory bodies and clinicians.

Institutional work comprises exactly these kinds of processes wherein seemingly irreconcilable or ethically complex issues are to be addressed and translated into legal and regulatory frameworks and clinical practices. In addition, institutional work needs to align the views and opinions of expert communities, in this case the professional community of reproductive medicine researchers and clinicians, and more lay communities that formally speaking have a say regarding regulatory issues. For instance, religious beliefs regarding the nature of family life and morals regarding sexuality have relatively little to do with the clinical work in IVF clinics. Yet lesbian couples, in a way deviating from traditional norms regarding family arrangements and therefore allegedly creating concerns regarding the interests and well-being of "the unborn child," were excluded from IVF therapies for more than two decades. Similarly, single women could not be legally fertilized until July 2015 in Sweden, a country that frequently takes pride in its work to create gender equality. The mismatch and difficulties involved in aligning biomedical research work and wider social interest and beliefs emphasizes the need for skillful institutional work wherein different views and interests are reconciled or at least temporarily harmonized into functional regulatory frameworks and practices.

Case 2: Pre-implantation genetic diagnosis and screening

Looking back at the development of ART, the clinical practices in the clinics were in many ways dependent on the advances of the field of reproductive medicine conducted in research university departments. This dependency existed both since the research expertise and resources were available in the university context and since the university researchers were granted the right to conduct research work that otherwise would have been complicated to get approval for. However, there was by no means a straightforward or linear relationship between the university departments and clinics. The interviewed researchers were well informed about clinical concerns and issues, and some of the private IVF clinics had a tradition of conducting research work as being part of their history from the early days of ART when the boundaries between the research universities and the clinics were quite vague and porous. For instance, one of the entrepreneurs in the IVF industry and a representative of the largest Scandinavian assisted reproduction company expressed his willingness to continue to support the strong research tradition in one of their clinics:

> When we acquired [a prestigious private clinic], having this solid research tradition, we started to discuss how we would handle this research issue, how to explore this tradition and make it beneficial for the entire concern. We then had this idea of creating a research company.
>
> (Entrepreneur, Ph.D. in Reproductive Medicine)

At the same time, the entrepreneur admitted that the research they planned should aim for "immediate results that benefit the patients." "Everything that can improve the results and enhance the treatment. That category of projects is in our interests," he said. One such domain of clinical research being of practical and short-term interests is to participate in clinical trials of new candidate drugs. In one of the clinics, many of the midwives had participated in such research projects and the outcome was that "there has been many new drugs and new therapies during the years we have been in operation" (Entrepreneur, Ph.D. in Reproductive Medicine).

Turning to the community of university-based researchers in disciplines such as gynecology, obstetrics, embryology research, and cytology, all contributing to reproductive medicine, they too were committed to the betterment of the existing methods and technologies. For instance, when asked what was ongoing "promising research" that was either of clinical relevance or interesting in a mid- to long-term perspective, one of the professors argued that the methods to reduce the hormone stimulation in women would be a prioritized domain of research. The professor remarked that Asian women in particular, being "small and lean" were overrepresented in hormone overstimulation cases, often being a condition demanding hospitalization and at times even being a life-threatening condition. The private assisted reproduction entrepreneur explained some of the undesirable side effects of the present hormone therapies:

> Previously, there was this treatment … giving menopause-like side-effects. That part [of the therapy] had very poor reputation. If you could substitute that with another model that did not give these side-effects and if you could shorten the period [of hormone stimulation], then much would have been won in terms of fewer side-effects and a higher degree of willingness to undergo the therapy again, if needed.
>
> (Entrepreneur, Ph.D. in Reproductive Medicine)

The professor in turn argued that a long-term objective was to "develop the egg in a media outside of the body" (Professor and reproductive medicine researcher, University Hospital, Sweden), reducing the hormone therapy to an absolute minimum. In her mind, much of the unwanted side effects from ineffective hormone therapies were largely unaccounted for in terms of social and individual costs, not least in the suffering of women being overstimulated: "You are concerned about how these women suffer, but there is no value of that calculated under these conditions," she said (Professor and reproductive medicine researcher, University Hospital, Sweden).

In addition to the more short-term practical research objectives, there was interrelated research interest in the field of reproductive medicine research that was bound up with, for instance, stem cell research, one of the principal scientific spin-offs from reproductive medicine. In the professor of reproductive medicine's research team, a method for establishing embryonal stem cell lines from biopsied single blastomeres from three-day old embryos had been successfully developed. The new method did not in any way harm or damage the embryo but the embryos could be transferred to the womb and develop into a fetus. The main contribution to the field of stem cell research is that one of the most heavily criticized features of the research work – its consumption of donated human embryos – would no longer be an important input material for the stem cell research practice.

Another field of ongoing research work was to better understand male infertility. One of the Ph.D. candidates being supervised by the professor used skin cells from patients with Kleinefelt's syndrome, leading to the inability to produce sperm, to better understand the biological pathways and mechanisms inhibiting male fertility. This research project was still in its infancy but testifies to the interest in male infertility on a broader basis. Similarly, the researchers noted a lack of research regarding the implantation of embryos and factors stemming from the uterus, due to a fixation on studying embryos and egg cells:

> What has been repeated over and over is that we examine the egg and embryos in IVF and so forth, but that there is a need for exploring the uterus. There is research in that area. The issue: How is the receptivity of the uterus? Can you increase the receptivity, and so forth?
>
> (Professor #2, reproductive medicine)

Social and cultural factors counteracted the advances of ART as especially middle-class, urban women tended to postpone parenting until their late 30s, clinicians argued. As a consequence, the success rate of the clinics were lowered by women in the age closer to 40 than 35 and there was a need for new clinical methods to better understand how previously supposedly fertile women gradually lose their reproductive capacities as they grow older. One such method that held a promise for better understanding was pre-implantation genetic diagnosis (PGD) and pre-implantation genetic screening (PGS). As the interviewees used the term PGS, we will stick to that acronym in the following, but remind the reader that these two terms are complicated to distinguish.

In the most research intensive of the private IVF companies, there was an initiative to conduct a larger research project aiming at making PGS a standard method for identifying genetic deviation in the embryos to be able to explain successive failed assisted reproduction therapies. The problem is that the general opinion and especially the political representatives that influenced regulatory decision tended to associate the use of PGD and PGS with a form of genetic engineering and an undesirable "eugenic medicine" where certain embryos could be eliminated. Speaking broadly about the "dignity of human life" and again what is "natural," some groups and decision-makers were very concerned about the consequences of PGS. A private company representative largely thought these objections were legitimate but that they overrated abstract and speculative risks at the expense of the practical utility of the methods:

> [The research project] has the purpose of enhancing the possibilities for those who passed through several treatment cycles but that have failed despite having fine embryos. Then you can make a test and conduct a genetic analysis. Studies abroad show that the embryos that looks good may be genetically defect. So it is a matter of identifying whether it [the embryo] is okay or if there are concerns that make it useless to transfer ... That would help many patients having a hard time to get helped by IVF: older women, recurrent failed treatment cycles, and miscarriages, these three cases.
>
> (Entrepreneur, Ph.D. in Reproductive Medicine)

The use of PGS without permission from the so-called Medical Ethics Review Board is illegal. The company thus had to design a research project and apply for the license to use PGS within a limited and controlled set of patients and embryos, and by the time of the interview, this research project was just about to be launched. For the private company, a new method to better select what embryos to not transfer may enhance the success rate of treatment cycles. As the private clinics to a larger extent received couples where the would-be mother was older than in the public clinics, or couples that had already been through a number of unsuccessful treatment cycles, the private clinics were eager to develop new methods. This ambition included not only the ability to understand and decode the significance of massive data sets of genetic information, but also to advance a change in public opinion and legal and regulatory changes. The entrepreneurs did not sweep the latter concern under the carpet but admitted frankly that they foresaw a change in the law: "We want to make clear that in the case of this method [the use of PGS], our goal is to accomplish a change of the law, quite simply. It is unreasonable that Sweden has a legislation that deviates from other [countries]" (Entrepreneur, Ph.D. in Reproductive Medicine).

Private IVF company representatives saw PGS as a new tool that could both enhance the precision of the therapy and that could be added as a service offered to clients. The administrator of an IVF company recognized the possibilities: "PGS is possible to sell as a separate service. It is quite expensive, actually. I think many would ask for it and pay for it as a separate service. That is how it works abroad today." In order to participate in this new domain of expertise, the IVF company had started a research project, a major investment for the firm, also including the hiring of a genetics researcher, a new professional category in the company:

> There are studies conducted [about the use of PGS] and this is regarded to be the next major shift happening. It is forbidden in Sweden today, precisely because there are not too many studies conducted to date. Ours is a big study: We have hired a geneticist and we have invested in very advanced technology. It will be a two to three years project ... You examine the chromosomes to identify deviations, because the conjecture is that the [embryo] do not stick [to the endometrium in the womb], quite simple.
>
> (CEO, IVF Company)

A representative of a company selling a new form of incubator including a camera incubator that provided a series of photographs of how the embryo develops over the period it is stored in the laboratory, also understood PGD as a method that competed with their product. PGS provided more precise genetic information about the embryo and thus complemented the visual inspection:

> There will be other screening methods which we will compete against, such as PGS. In at least the US but also in other markets, that is connected with a nice income for the doctors, so we have to convince them that you can get similar information – not the same, but similar information – from the incubator [camera] at a lower cost level. And then it's up to the doctor how he can market it and then still get the profit. But that's absolutely something going on in the PGS market as well.
>
> (Chief Commercial Officer, Medical Technology Firm)

If permitted on a broader basis, PGS would open up new clinical and commercial possibilities. By and large, which may be somewhat surprising or counterintuitive, the private clinics were willing to invest a substantial share of their profits in new research projects. The PGS project was one such investment, but the private company also tried out new tools, such as the private company representatives said, "syringes that hurt less when procuring the eggs" (Entrepreneur, Ph.D. in Reproductive Medicine). Besides adding to the quality of the therapies, participation in such research work served to motivate the clinic staff: "To develop the practices creates a sense of confidence, and it is research work that after all really can change this industry" (Entrepreneur, Ph.D. in Reproductive Medicine).

However, resistance to PGS/PGD at the level of policy-makers and health care provider administrators was described as common among our interviewees. Offering publicly financed PGD to couples with rare genetic diseases had been discussed, said one politician, yet the advantages of using IVF and screening the embryos were weighed against the possibility of this new treatment opening up to further additional new treatments. Prioritizing one group of patients before others was seen as difficult:

> We also had a discussion, there is a disease where you have a sick baby. Many women have to go through several abortions, because you can't see if the baby is sick until after a while [during the pregnancy]. Then you could instead do a test-tube fertilization really, take out the egg and check if it is healthy before ... that then becomes one of these issues: 'if we say yes to this, then they have been allowed to be prioritized [instead of others]'.
>
> (Regional politician in the area of health care)

The politician explained that individual professionals working in the related area of health care typically were important in implementing new methods. The politicians were often the ones resisting ideas of investing or raising costs and thought the developments were too new and untested:

> I guess it is a general rule that I have learned after my time in this job, when it comes to implementation of new health care methods: that it is in the hands of one or two persons. It normally is with one head physician, who takes it way too far, in other words they want to be too early and too expensive. That's what is normal. A head physician has something new that they want to try because it develops their job.
>
> (Regional politician in the area of health care)

However, when it came to PGS the politician suspected that the reasons for not allowing it or including it as part of the public health care at IVF clinics were not mainly to do with public finances. The opponents of implementing this new technology used irrational arguments and scare tactics, according to the interviewee:

> And my worry and suspicion is that there are, if not religious, then at least stale and old values that are irrational, that are directing the actions in this area./.../ Like in the PGS debate they use scare tactics, 'this isn't safe, the outcome isn't really good.' They scare with genes. Some politicians tremble when they hear the word genetic diagnosing. Despite that we use the exact same genetic diagnosing, in different ways today.
>
> (Regional politician in the area of health care)

The resistance to PGS and similar new technologies in health care did not follow any particular political ideologies or party lines. It was instead described as a personal or generational view that colored the position of politicians debating new IVF technologies and treatments. Younger generations take the technologies more for granted, thought the politician:

> But in this specific area there is some kind of difference of values where there is a conservative line which isn't really about the political scale, but it is very much up to each person what your view is on both infertility treatment and other issues of the crotch ... Possibly, one could say that this is a generational and age related question. In the sense that many of the so-called newfangled developments that have come in this area are seen as staple food for those who did not live in a time when it wasn't around. For those who live in a reality where we have children later and later, and you have many friends that have struggled with this, then it isn't something you are against. It's the opposite; you demand to be helped.
>
> (Regional politician working in the area of health care)

Thus, the use of PGD or PGS in public IVF health care in Sweden was debated, while being offered under restrictions in private clinics. In the policy domain, new technologies such as these were often proposed and supported by head physicians, but were judged by policy-makers based on cost–benefit analysis. Their analysis was also described as being dependent on the general acceptance of IVF and new genetic technologies.

Case 3: The uterus transplantation project

In comparison to PGD and PGS, being based on by now widely established genomics methods and de facto being in operation to identify some genetic deviations at an early stage including Down's syndrome, the uterus transplantation project located at the Sahlgrenska Medical Academy at the University of Gothenburg was far more innovative and visionary. The project was also riddled by uncertainty and again a fair share of skepticism from individuals concerned about the legitimacy and practical consequences of too far-reaching interventions into the human reproductive capacities. The Sahlgrenska Academy has a long tradition of research in reproductive medicine and was the site of the birth of the fourth IVF baby in the world and the first in Scandinavia. Since the late 1970s, many clinical studies have been conducted at the medical school, demonstrating the safety and efficacy of assisted reproduction.

Today, in the middle of the second decade of the new millennium, close to four decades after the birth of the first baby fertilized in the laboratory, the Sahlgrenska Academy hosts a unique uterus transplantation project, a research project where women born without a uterus, or who have lost it through injuries or illness, have this organ transplanted from living donors (in many cases the mothers of the recipients) to be able to give birth to a baby in the future. The project is a combination of reproductive medicine and organ transplant medicine. The principal investigator, a professor in gynecology, told the story that led to his interest in accomplishing this visionary objective, starting in Australia where the professor was working for a period of time:

> Back in 1998, I was working in Australia. I operated on this woman for cervix cancer, she was 25, very charismatic, beautiful woman that I had to do a radical hysterectomy on. I said to her: 'Your ovaries are in place and your hormone, but your uterus is gone, so you cannot become a mother.' 'But cannot you transplant a uterus?' [she responded]. I had not thought of the possibility of doing that. I thought she was slightly mental. But after a while, the idea did not sound too strange.
>
> (Professor #2, reproductive medicine)

While the professor admitted that the surgery involved was "complicated" and that there were possibly no more than 2,000 women in Sweden (having a population around 9.5 million) that would be the principal beneficiaries of the research work, he still thought this was one method to further enable human fertility. "Uterus transplantation is a small field. There are perhaps ten research teams being active in the world, in the U.S., Australia, Japan, Europe," the professor explained. Out of the total amount of eleven successful uterus transplantations, nine had been conducted in Gothenburg. In addition, most of the patients have responded to the surgery much better than was predicted and no patients had any major complications to date. Unfortunately, the research shows that the ovaries being donated may not "have the quality we hoped for," the professor claimed. For the time being, it was yet to be seen whether the women receiving uteruses would be able to become mothers.

The surgery conducted quite recently followed ten years of minute preparations, including transplanting uteruses of mice, pigs, sheep and eventually many trips to Kenya where the project team could train to transfer uteruses from primates. The story of how the project team learned the practical work to conduct the transplantation surgery reveals that there were enormous practical issues to be handled in every stage of the work. The anesthesiologist of the uterus transplantation research team explained how the project received ethical permissions to operate on larger animals but under the conditions that the animals should live, thereby creating the concern on how to anesthesize animals and how to determine signs of pain: "How can you identify pain in an animal? They do not signal their pain in the same manner. If they limp, they limp, but it is not that they yell or anything. We're not that different, thank God! ... Animals also get nervous, so how can you handle them without making them terrified?" (Anesthesiologist, Uterus Transplantation Research Program). By and large, the animals operated on were treated just like human patients, under normal conditions subject to strict regulations and policies:

> The pigs were anesthesized. They were terrified, more so than a human would be. They are subject to intubation, that is you place this tube into their throat. When being on the operation table, they should be comfortable and there cannot be any pressure wounds. Well, you know. All these concerns! They cannot be too cold. They must sleep well and receive the same kind of pain relief ... It is the same machines, the same respirators.
>
> (Anesthesiologist, Uterus
> Transplantation Research Program)

Later on, the project included primates to provide surgery experience in a specimen more closely resembling humans. "Monkeys are terrifyingly fascinating – they look just like us on the inside, but there is less fat. The proportions are also smaller," the anesthesiologist said. In this phase, the anesthesiologist work became even more complicated as there was only limited know-how among zoologists regarding how to handle the monkeys both during the surgery and in the post-operation process. "The monkeys, they were an entirely new thing, you can say … There's no one anesthesizing monkeys in Sweden. A few times [in the zoos] where they conduct cesarean births at times" (Anesthesiologist, Uterus Transplantation Research Program). After the surgery was conducted, the post-operation phase also proved to be challenging:

> Monkeys are complicated to handle in the post-operation phase because they live in communities. They constantly defend their social ranking in the community. If they are taken away from the community, they will fight their way back in when they return. And then they won't demonstrate any signs of weakness, like pain. And they remove everything you put on them, like syringes.
>
> (Anesthesiologist, Uterus
> Transplantation Research Program)

Despite all the practical issues to handle and the ordeal, the anesthesiologist described the ten-year period as being intellectually stimulating and he appreciated being part of something new and innovative:

> The best part has been that we had a good time and enjoyed our work and that we have been able to enter worlds none of us knew existed. It's been a great time! What else? There are new ideas emerging all the time. We have entered a new world of thought. In addition, we need to learn how to handle the quite practical problems, the patients. The negative part is that it has taken such a long time.
>
> (Anesthesiologist, Uterus
> Transplantation Research Program)

Once being able to master the transplant surgery in primates, the team moved on to recruit patients and donors in Sweden. Under all conditions, the whole procedure includes a series of very complicated surgical operations and careful analyses of how the patients respond to the surgery: "There is so much hard work. It is not only a matter of operating, but all these things afterwards and before, and so forth" (Professor #2, reproductive medicine). He continued to explain the sheer work time needed to complete the entire surgery, including not one but two patients:

It is so damn hard! … Just look at the operation times here: Anesthesia, time to produce the specimen – twelve hours and thirty-seven minutes … That was the procurement … But you also need to transplant it … that takes five to six hours. It is a difficult operation.

(Professor #2, reproductive medicine)

The anesthesiologist said that "it was a more complicated surgery work than we expected." The timetables for the surgery derived from the primate operations were not predicting the actual surgery operation time at all, and e.g., to retrieve the womb, "that took so much longer time than in the monkeys," the anesthesiologist argued:

We had practiced for such a long time. In regular hysterectomy you cut off the blood vessels close to the womb [this is not the case in transplant surgery]. And you need to be very careful with the ureters and the nerves and all that. Still, we were surprised about the complexity of the surgery.

(Anesthesiologist, Uterus
Transplantation Research Program)

"The first two patients were really no routine job. But after three, four, five, I'd say that it all fell into place. We developed a routine," the anesthesiologist said.

The actual surgery work aside, there are also a series of medical issues that need to be carefully monitored, including the complication of immunosuppression, the damage of the vessels in the uterus and the surrounding tissue, a factor that may prove uterus transplant surgery ineffective as a method to handle infertility, the professor admitted:

What speaks against [the transplantation] is the surgery … There's been a trauma in the uterus and the vessels, the *immunosuppression*. We know that the immunosuppression … increases the risks for deformations, increases the risks for miscarriages, and so forth ... What speaks in favour of it is that there are some women that get pregnant quite easily, so some should get pregnant here as well. But we do not know yet ... if we start with nine women, I do not think there will be nine mothers. But hopefully three or four.

(Professor #2, reproductive medicine. Emphasis in the original)

Prior to any transfer of embryos – subject to assisted reproduction in the laboratory – the uterus has to stabilize for more than a year within the body. The professor continued:

The transplants are done, but we cannot transfer the embryos until a year later ... There have been evidence of early pregnancies leading to miscarriages, and the goal is actually to be the first one to give birth to a baby. That would be the definition of a successful transplantation. The uterus being in place and the ovulation working, that is one thing, but that is not the goal. No one in the world has yet accomplished this objective.

(Professor #2, reproductive medicine)

It demands no detailed expertise in surgery and medicine to realize the complexity of the pursuit to first transfer a uterus between two women and thereafter produce a pregnancy in the transferred womb; there are high risks involved and the costs at these early stages are not negligible. Not least there are expertise, skills, and know-how dedicated to the project that possibly could have been used better elsewhere, the critics claim. The professor was of course highly informed about all kinds of objections and critiques, but he constantly received letters of interest and encouraging notes from childless women and couples, supporting his belief in the importance of the uterus transfer project. Like in many other cases, the closest and adjacent professional disciplines hosted the most ardent skeptics:

The largest skepticism is encountered here, in this very building we are working. [The] reproductive medicine [department] has been quite skeptical ... We have received quite much media attention, not so much in Sweden but we have been in CNN and BBC News ... so there's been some attention. But there is little recognition in our own organization. But that's life!

(Professor #2, reproductive medicine)

Writing off skepticism to some extent as being an envious response to the struggle over resources and jurisdictional claims, there was still the ethical issue of where to draw the boundary between what could be legitimately conducted on the basis of scientific interests in the field of human reproduction. Moreover, the allocation of health care budgets was another concern, where different therapies and policies were pitted, as always, against one another. The politicians that we interviewed attested to this view, that procedures to alleviate infertility were sometimes discussed as less important, compared to other types of health care:

> There are other things that we have taken out of our offering, like plastic surgery and other things. If we go in that direction, when you say that this isn't a life-threatening condition, it isn't a disease ... Then it is more an issue, well of course it is a disease or what you should call it, it is a condition where you are not reproductive. But you can live well with it, it isn't a threat.
>
> (Health care administrator for a regional government body)

Yet, following the developments and being ready to change decisions is important, when it comes to controversial treatments, he explained. The developments are happening so quickly, decisions cannot be set in stone but are always weighed in terms of costs and benefits:

> We politicians are humans too. I believe that the changes in society and the development is moving so quickly, so I think that everyone feels that all decisions can't be set in stone ... Particularly these somewhat more controversial things, you have to be ready to do a follow-up and see what happens, should we change our minds, should we take another step? It can be an issue of costs sometimes. /.../ IVF in total isn't any big cost in our budget./.../ If we go back, I think it has maybe more been seen as a luxury issue 'Should we really pay for it?' and so on.
>
> (Regional politician working in health care)

The professor working on developing the technology of uterus transplantations tried to muddle through such an archipelago of criticism and practical concerns and justified the work of his research team as being an innovative way to combine domains of medical and surgical expertise to accomplish new and previously unseen methods.

Also in this case, the stem cell technology being developed from within reproductive medicine, embryology, and cytology, was a factor to consider. In one of the more visionary speculations about what would possibly happen in the field in the future, the professor addressed the challenge to find live donors that were willing to spare their wombs. If a uterus could be harvested from a human cadaver, it could be combined with stem cell technologies to avoid the recipient's body refusing the new organ:

> The concept is to procure a uterus from a cadaver and remove all cells so you have a scaffold and this three-dimensional architecture. You take the patient's own stem cells to build an organ [on the scaffold] and then you can return it to the patient to avoid a transplant rejection. You reduce the surgical risks … and there is an unlimited source of organs.
>
> (Professor #2, reproductive medicine)

This procedure would first make the supply of organs virtually unlimited, compared to that there are relatively few women that suffer from the medical condition who want to become parents, and are willing to undergo the surgery demanded. Second, it would reduce the surgery operation time as there is merely one patient to operate on, leading to less demanding work on the part of the surgery team. The professor was again fully aware of the common sense critique of the scenario of harvesting a uterus from a cadaver and growing stem cells on the scaffold to thereafter transplant the uterus into a woman, in turn giving birth to a baby. Such transgressions across the life/death divide would certainly move beyond ideas regarding "what life admits" and "what is natural." Fortunately (for some) and unfortunately (for others), not all researchers and clinical practitioners pledge their allegiance to such beliefs but take on the role to actively explore the boundaries for what human medical technoscience may enable, leading to new practices that extend beyond the limits of common sense thinking. The uterus transplantation project certainly rests on such ambitions.

Summary and conclusion

Institutional work aimed at creating new possibilities and, in the long-term perspective, new institutions, in many cases encounters the stern resistance of common sense thinking. Not only the proverbial "wo/man on the street" can be strongly opinionated about biomedical matters and controversies but also regulators and representatives of policy-making bodies ground their decisions in inherited norms and values, in many cases leading to the instinctual response to block or counteract any social change. As Sigmund Freud remarked, change, no matter how positive, always requires expenditures of mental energy and demands acts of adaptation, both asking for more from the individual than he or she may be willing to give. In cases where decision-making and policy-making are scrutinized by others, this instinctual resistance to change needs to be balanced by more rational lines of reasoning. Under all conditions, institutional work is what is beset by skepticism and concerns regarding quite abstract norms held in esteem, e.g., ideas about "human nature," its "dignity" and needs for being protected against external influences. At the same time, the wo/man on the street has historically demonstrated much faith in science and the work of scientists, at times to the level where such faith cannot be fully justified, so the modernist dream about a shining future accomplished on scientific expertise blends with an instinctual resistance to change in ways that are complicated to fully predict by e.g., policy-makers. In addition, the know-how and interest in reproductive medicine differs substantially across the population, with e.g., women demonstrating a somewhat higher degree of engagement, some interviewees suggest, adding to the complexity of the institutional work to create new practices. These conditions make institutional work a form of political game including professional groups, patients, regulators, and a number of additional stakeholders, all having their own interests and objectives.

6 Maintaining institutions

Pricing therapies and developing markets in the ART industry

Introduction

In the second of the three empirical chapters, the concept of institutional work aimed at maintaining existing institutions and practices will be addressed. As explained at the end of Chapter 2 in Part I of the book, institutional maintenance is the process wherein primarily insiders, i.e., professionals and experts, engage in upholding standard procedures for clinical practices, technologies, and processes that serve to provide stable access to treatments. In this chapter, two forms of institutional maintenance work will be examined: structuring the market and pricing the treatments. These two themes include the role of the state and the market, standardizing ART in a mature field, strategies for covering costs, the bidding process for contracts with the government, market penetration and investments abroad, the issue of medical tourism, how the market is made and the suppliers' view of this market.

ART in Sweden

The structure of the Swedish IVF market

Sweden has been at the forefront of reproductive medicine research and in the development of clinically assisted reproduction practices. Active research in follow-up studies of the new generation of babies fertilized conducted by Swedish research teams in the 1980s and 1990s have revealed that there are no differences between the naturally conceived babies and the babies fertilized in the laboratory; both groups of children demonstrate the same intellectual and emotional development trajectories. The Swedish reproductive medicine policy is structured around a concern for the unborn child, and in practice that means that a traditional nuclear family structure has been favored as the best family setting for children. As a consequence, lesbian couples were not made eligible for the treatment until 2006, after more than two decades of clinical operations, and single women are still not eligible for the therapy.

In the post-World War II period, Sweden has politically favored a "third-way politics" agenda, including a combination of a substantial public sector and private initiatives but has slowly moved towards more market liberal policies. In the specific case of assisted reproduction therapies, this means that the first born child can be fertilized in a public sector clinic (in many cases a private clinic working under a public sector contract), while siblings need to be paid for in privately owned and operated clinics (or in some cases by paying the full cost fee to a public clinic). The subsidized price paid by the client ("the patient") in the public sector treatment is a standardized health care fee of around 10 euros per visit, while the private full fee therapy costs around 33,000 Swedish crowns (around 4,000 euros). While this latter cost is significantly higher than the public sector fee, it is still a price that many families can afford and that is significantly lower than in e.g., the U.K. or the U.S.

Moreover, the Swedish public health care organizations are structured into regional organizations and into 20 health care regions (*Landsting*) having their own governing bodies including political representatives elected every fourth year. The regional health care organizations can independently make decisions regarding for instance the maximum age of eligible clients and there are some differences between parts of Sweden regarding the generosity of public sector reproductive health care. For instance, the northernmost region is renowned for being more strict (basically explained on the basis of a shrinking tax-payer base and a higher proportion of elderly to care for) on the age of the female clients than elsewhere as well as the number of attempts, and while there are recommendations from governmental agencies regarding for instance age limits, there is still some variation in the field.

The reproductive health care services provided by the public sector is a combination of clinics being part of the public sector, as in the case of the clinics located at the major university hospitals, and private clinics that are commissioned to provide the same services. The license to deliver IVF treatments to the public sector is earned in a bidding system wherein different private clinic and health care companies submit their applications to the regional health care organization's procurement offices. The bid includes both qualifying criteria and order-wining criteria, and in most cases it is the success rate of the therapies (measured as the ratio of reported pregnancies to the number of treatment cycles) and the price that are demanded. The procurement officers contracting the private clinics thus need to value the success rate in relation to the price to be paid, and in some cases the more efficient clinic may win the bid despite demanding a higher price.

The price paid for the private clinic services by the clients, either having one child already or being older than the age limits enacted by the regional health care organizations, derive from market-based pricing. In most cases, this means a cost-based pricing with a few extra percent to enable an operative profit to be generated. The contacts provided by the regional health care sectors are important for the private clinics for two reasons: First, all IVF clinics have substantial fixed costs that need to be covered, and profits in the operations can only be ensured after the nth client has paid for their treatments. That is, the clinics are dependent on relatively high volumes. In addition to cost coverage derived from the use of highly skilled staff and advanced technologies, the professional co-workers demand a certain workload to maintain and further develop their skills. Second, as the public sector health care organization provides therapies for only the first-born child, creating contacts with clients during the first treatments and pregnancies increases the chances of attracting returning clients. Being granted the license to operate within the public sector health organization thus adds valuable marketing opportunities for the private clinics.

While this system may not be perfect, it still offers some advantages for the three categories of actors (public sector health care organization, the private clinics, and the clients). The public sector organization benefits from taking advantage of the expertise and know-how developed in the private clinics, while the bidding system serves to counteract a too high cost for the tax-funded health care sector. The private clinics need to report their formal performance data and the calculated price they demand to deliver the service, so they need to constantly further develop their clinical skills and day-to-day operations. In the case of private clinics winning the contract, they get a stable stock of clients that cover fixed costs or in some cases contribute to generating a profit, and they are likely to take advantage of returning clients. The clients, finally, can take advantage of world-class expertise at first a comparatively low cost, and if they are successful in becoming parents, they can return to pay a higher price for the second child in a clinic they are already familiar with.

There are constant debates and discussions regarding how much the public sector should invest in infertility treatment vis-à-vis other health care therapies, and some critics argue that assisted reproduction is a form of "luxury medicine" that should not be included in the public health care offering. On the other hand, infertility and childlessness are documented sources of individual suffering and social costs, and it has been calculated that the economic benefits for society investing in IVF therapies are substantial. These benefits derive from both reduced health care costs for depressed individuals failing to become parents, and the calculated future tax income generated by the child born as a result of IVF technology. In fact, many representatives of the field suggest that Sweden should pursue an even more generous legislation on the basis of such data, making e.g., single women eligible for the therapy. As in many other cases, the public health care sector needs to balance a variety of interests and objectives reasonably well, and the present system seems to balance e.g., private and public initiatives, cost-pressure and innovation, and pursue egalitarian values as all families can at least have their first-born child fertilized in the laboratory. In the following, empirical data will be reported, indicating how the public sector bidding system contributes to making the activities more efficient at the same time as there is room for profits in the private clinics that can be reinvested to further strengthen the expertise and technological standard of the clinics.

Reaching maturity: consequences of ART becoming standardized

Like in many other knowledge-intensive and science-based industries, the key to long-term competitiveness is to recruit and motivate skilled professionals that can be in charge of the operations. As IVF has gradually matured and become a standard therapy, there are both less controversies and animated debates regarding the technoscientific and medical intervention into the elementary processes of human reproduction, but there is also a decline of the attractiveness of the therapeutic area, some of the interviewees argued.

Twenty years ago, the situation looked quite different, when "reproductive medicine was on top" (Professor #2, reproductive medicine) of the medical fields. The retiring generation of professors in reproductive medicine was also served the dual role of being the entrepreneurs that started the first private clinics in Stockholm and Gothenburg, while there was no equally ambitious and entrepreneurial generation ready to take their place. This was described as leading to a downward spiral in both the university setting and in the industry. One important factor to consider when explaining this decline is the absence of funding, possibly rooted in the enactment of reproductive medicine as what is not a fully legitimate professional sub-field within medicine, stretching back to the 1950s and 1960s when reproductive medicine was mobilized to handle the escalating overpopulation problem.

In addition, another professor in reproductive medicine claimed that the lack of qualified leadership skills in the university setting serves to de-motivate the research community, who are increasingly burdened by various administrative tasks and managerial initiatives that add little to the actual research work:

> The leadership skills are underdeveloped in this field ... There should be more possibilities for clinical research work than is the case today ... to be able to reduce the risks and in the future be able to offer IVF without using all these expensive hormones.
>
> (Professor, reproductive medicine,
> University Hospital, Sweden)

The challenge for the field of academic reproductive medicine both benefitted the private clinics and was one of their concerns. On the positive account, the loss of attraction of the academic research career made it easier to recruit skilled clinicians. On the other hand, the lack of progress in the academic research work rendered reproductive medicine marginal and made it a somewhat dull, run-of-the-mill field of research, piping research talent into other domains of medical research. One way to handle this downturn in attractiveness was that the private clinics did their best to initiate and host research work. In one large company this was organized as a separate non-profit subsidiary, which made it possible to receive donations by e.g. pharmaceutical companies:

> The research company is a non-profit company. The business concern has a parent company and a number of subsidiaries. The research company is one of several subsidiaries, having its own articles of association, that prevents it from reporting profits to the parent company...That was a key issue to handle, because no one would be willing to donate money to a research company in a private concern where they risk that the money ends up as profits in the parent company.
>
> (Entrepreneur, Ph.D. in Reproductive Medicine)

At the same time, operating in an environment characterized by a high degree of regulations and fierce cost pressure made it complicated for the private clinics to uphold this image of "dynamic research sites," one of the professors argued:

> There is always this attempt to look really research intense, but there is not much going on [in the clinics]. There is one clinic conducting much research in Sweden. They have plowed down quite a bit of research in their R&D activities, but I suppose it is not a major activity. On the other hand, there is not much going on in reproductive medicine at all, for the time being.
>
> (Professor #2, reproductive medicine)

While there were in fact many new challenges, both scientific and clinical, to be handled, for instance, the qualities of embryos selected and the uses of PGS technologies to understand infertility, there were still some concerns regarding the future of the research work in the new situation where assisted reproduction has become a staple method of medicine. Both public sector and private organizations struggled to create possibilities for attracting skilled co-workers.

The pricing of assisted reproduction services: the role of the state and the market

Running the clinic and covering the costs

Among the interviewees, there was no major critique of the Swedish system to combine public sector clinics and private clinics to provide qualified health care services at a reasonable cost. One of the representatives of a private clinic company saw many benefits in the existing system:

> I really do believe in a combination of private and public health care. Many IVF treatments are today conducted in the private sector, but financed by tax money. They have smaller units, work more effectively, and you get more for the money.
>
> (Resident Surgery and Gynecology,
> Medical director, Private Clinic Company)

There were relatively few co-workers in the private clinics that did not have any background in medicine and health care, and the industry representatives were by and large more concerned about offering high qualitative therapies and further developing the clinical practices than extracting short-term profits from the clinics. However, one of the key financial objectives for the clinics was to cover their fixed costs. In practice, this means that each clinic needs to report between 400 and 500 treatment cycles annually to secure an operative profit. Says one of the private clinic representatives:

A clinic conducting less than 500 treatment cycles [annually] would not be able to carry its own costs. So you need something like 500 to 1,000 treatment cycles. You cannot run a clinic below the costs of 20 million [Swedish] crowns, I believe.

(Entrepreneur, Ph.D. in Reproductive Medicine)

In addition, another private clinic representative similarly estimated the need for approximately 400 treatment cycles annually:

A private clinic is financed by the patients and that they pay for their investigations and their treatment. You need these 400 treatment cycles. That is a break-even point, so to speak. The costs for the laboratory staff, the media you use, the IVF therapy. I cannot say exactly what those costs are today, but a few years back, when I was working in a smaller clinic, we calculated that it would costs around 15,000 crowns for one treatment cycle.

(Resident Surgery and Gynecology,
Medical director, Private IVF Company)

At the same time as there is much concern for covering the fixed costs every fiscal year, the private IVF clinics have historically been very profitable. The CFO of one private ART company owning a series of clinics in Sweden said the operative profit was in the 20 to 30 percent range. Also the first private clinics started in the 1980s were profitable "from day one," as one private clinic representative recalled.

This ability to report significant levels of profit, a standard economic theory argument proposes, would attract investors from outside the industry. While there are stories told about certain private clinics located in the major cities being contacted by venture capital firms every now and then, the privately owned Swedish assisted reproduction clinics are still today, after three decades of operations, run mainly by physicians with a background in reproductive medicine, gynecology, cytology, embryology and similar disciplines immediately related to the clinical practice. A large IVF company with several clinics is partly owned by an investment fund that raises money for charitable causes; their investment is long term, the CEO explained. Rather than pursuing short-term value extraction strategies to maximize the financial gains of the owners, a substantial share of the profits have been reinvested in either clinical research or in new technologies such as modern incubators.

In order to cover fixed costs, the private clinics were willing to accept contracts where the economic compensation per treatment cycle was not very favorable, at times barely covering fixed costs, but the economic benefits for the clinic were still larger that calculated the costs: "The contract we have with [one health care region] are not very beneficial financially for us. But we become known and the patients who get a child may return for siblings. It is always good to be visible" (CFO, Private IVF company). More importantly for the clients, the public sector bidding system, enacted by the Swedish Public Sector Procurement Act, served the more indirect role of keeping the prices in the private clinics relatively low.

Many of the industry representatives took pride in not charging unreasonable prices to the clients: "In comparison to e.g., legal services, we do not at all ask for proper compensation," said one interviewee (Resident Surgery and Gynecology, Medical director, Private IVF company). He continued: "IVF is extremely cheap in Sweden in comparison to the U.S. The cost is roughly four times higher [in the U.S.]. In the U.K. – twice the price. And they do not report better results. Quite the contrary!" The CFO of the private company pointed at the price increases over the last 25 years in fact being lower than the average consumer price index: "When I started here in 1988, the IVF therapy cost 25,000 crowns, and today it costs 33,000 crowns. But that is 25 years later!," she exclaimed.

In an international comparison, the Swedish policy was to provide the clients with a fixed price for a certain treatment, a pricing model that was not used in e.g., the U.K. This is more transparent and fair to the clients, the CFO of a private IVF company argued:

> In an international perspective, we have quite low prices. We received a few patients from the UK, for instance, to our clinics, and in the UK and the US, this is more of a business, generally speaking. What clients appreciate is that in Sweden, the price agreed upon is the price you pay. In England ... [clients] are quite critical about the profession as they sell you additional treatments all the time, which the patient has a hard time to evaluate. If the physicians say, 'I believe we better do another ultrasound check here. That'll be 200 pounds,' it is really hard for the patient to say, 'No, I think we better save that money' when being told to do so by the doctor. So even though the list price is the same in Sweden as in the UK, when you leave the clinic you have paid the double or the triple.
>
> (CEO, Assisted reproduction company)

So, taken together, the Swedish private–public collaboration in assisted conception health care work benefits from both stability and long-term growth; the prices are reasonable as the sheer amount of demand ensures that the private clinics can run at substantial profit levels. At the same time, the community-based culture of the assisted reproduction industry has raised entry barriers for e.g., venture capital firms, and as a consequence, the private clinics are still today, when entering a more mature phase, primarily owned and managed by individuals with a background in health care and reproductive medicine, sharing the commitment to deliver high-quality therapies and to finance new development work.

The bidding process

A key issue in maintaining a competitive and dynamic IVF industry is to ensure that the bidding process is not violated by forms of opportunistic behavior, enabling less qualified but cheaper operators to win contracts from the public sector health care organization. The representatives of the private clinics described the relationship between the public and the private clinics as being "quite fine" as there were ongoing exchanges of co-workers and expertise between the clinics:

> The relationship to the public clinics, I think it is quite fine ... We try to maintain good relations. That is important, because we recruit our co-workers from there. At times, the relationship is being burdened when too many are being recruited from one single clinic at the same time.
>
> (Entrepreneur, Ph.D. in Reproductive Medicine)

It is important to remember that the professional field of reproductive medicine and its clinical branch, assisted reproduction, is quite small, and that most people know each other, making this a close-knit community of experts and co-workers. Physicians specializing in reproductive medicine and gynecology were particularly favored by the limited supply of expertise in the area, and recruitment between clinics was therefore always a delicate matter. As a consequence, the private clinic representatives tried their best to maintain good relations with the public sector health care organization: "We do collaborate with the regional health care organizations, but you don't dare to mess with them too much," one CEO (Private IVF company) argued. However, this willingness to maintain harmonious relations and to endorse a "live and let live" attitude was put to the test when new contracts were negotiated and when bids were issued. In such periods, politics tended to enter the otherwise stable relations. Formally speaking, the process was quite transparent in what information should be disclosed in the application:

> It looks a little bit different [in different health care regions]. In most cases, you have these formal demands that need to be fulfilled. And then you have the order-winning criteria being graded. Those are the quality parameters. Treatment results are the most important criteria. And then you add the prices the clients pay ... When you have placed your bid, the lowest price wins.
>
> (CEO, Assisted reproduction company)

In a few cases, there were bids from certain clinics being lower than most industry representatives thought were practically possible. The medical director of a private clinic addressed one such case:

> You also want more patients to get a more even and larger volume. That is good for the experience, to have many patients ... Our clinics in [a smaller town], they had this contract with a health care region, but then all of a sudden, there was another bid from a clinic outside of our company, asking for 10,000 [SEK] per treatment. They are not able to make the ends meet on that price, no chance! My guess is that they at least have to charge 15,000 to 20,000 per treatment cycle. 20,000 is actually what it costs. But they possibly needed these patients to get the volume. But then they dump the price for all

of us. In addition, the profits made are reinvested in the activities, to develop the work and to buy ultrasound technology, research work and so forth.

(Resident Surgery and Gynecology,
Medical director, Private IVF company)

In such cases, the clinic in question requires a larger stock of treatment cycles to break even, so they are perhaps willing to accept a lower price per cycle. But for many industry representatives, such pricing strategies was a violation of the widely agreed upon norm that one must not "dump the price" in order to gain short-term advantages. Such bidding tactics tend to conceal the actual costs. However, if a private clinic wins a contract on the basis of such procedures, being in the borderland of what is illegitimate behavior, the private clinics expect the public sector organization to actually stick to the formal agreement. At least in one case, interviewees referred to one example of how one private clinic had received higher economic compensation than prescribed in the contract, being clearly a deviation from Swedish public sector procurement law and the culture of the industry. Needless to say, this did not pass unrecognized in the industry:

> This was clearly a disgusting violation of the rules, because they have this contract and the price prescribed should be paid. Those are our terms, those are the term anyone else … I had heard these rumours … that [another private clinic] get paid twenty-one or twenty-two thousands [Swedish crowns] per treatment instead of the eighteen thousands they should receive. But I rest my case.

(CEO, Assisted reproduction company)

One may notice here that the CEO clearly did not want to rock the boat but was biding his time, being aware that both the private clinics benefitting from the additional compensation and the public sector organization representatives would know they had acted in culpable ways. Such a "stiff upper lip" attitude reveals both the willingness to maintain stable long-term relations in the industry and across the private–public boundaries, and the fact that the IVF company was still running at a solid profit. Incidents like the one described above are also exceptional cases, the interviews suggest, and a combination of professional ethics and norms and legal and regulatory control jointly keep such opportunistic behavior at bay.

In summary, the cost coverage, price-setting routines, and the formal bidding system are constitutive elements in the Swedish assisted reproduction industry, being at the forefront of efficiency and low prices for the clients. The public sector organization ensures that all Swedish citizens can take advantage of state-of-the-art expertise and technology, but also serve to push down the prices paid in the private clinics, basically using a cost-plus pricing policy. At the same time, the demand for IVF therapies are so voluminous, especially in the major cities, that most existing clinics are reporting stable levels of profit earnings. Public sector concerns for equality and equal rights to qualified health care and private sector venturing are thus arguably a recipe that has benefitted Swedish couples, paying a significantly lower price than e.g., their British and American counterparts.

Market penetration strategies: investing abroad

One way for the private IVF companies to expand their activities to increase their ability to cover fixed cost was to acquire clinics or companies abroad. The largest Swedish assisted reproduction company, running six clinics in Sweden, had enacted the strategy of investigating places to operate outside of Sweden. The founder claimed that when the company had acquired a number of clinics in Sweden, now being the only firm owning more than one clinic, the CEO was contacted by venture capital firms, a new group of investors in the field, now paying attention to the development in the IVF industry. While these contacts led nowhere at this point, it was apparent that the company now had a unique position in the Swedish market and that they might have the resources to exploit synergies in their operations. In Sweden, the market is both saturated and there may be anti-trust legislation on either national or the European level that may prohibit a further market penetration on the home market:

> It is so much easier to start a clinic in Sweden than abroad ... [but] I think there are few places in Sweden where one could compete with one additional clinic. I do not really know what the anti-trust legislation says. We are after all quite big.
>
> (Entrepreneur, Ph.D. in Reproductive Medicine)

Given these conditions, moving abroad would be the next step in the process: "We continue to grow but we can no longer grow in Sweden. We have to look for new markets ... We are really close [to a deal] in Poland. There's this chain of clinics that we have examined a number of times" (Entrepreneur, Ph.D. in Reproductive Medicine). In order to pursue a successful internationalization strategy, there are a number of factors that need to be fulfilled. First of all, the clinic acquired should be "up and running," having its own stock of clients and a reputation as a credible actor in the market:

> You look for established clinics, right. To be able to operate in another country, you need to buy an established, renowned clinic where everything works ... Using that as a platform, you can acquire other clinics in the country.
>
> (Entrepreneur, Ph.D. in Reproductive Medicine)

Second, there needs to be a shared view in the bidding company and the clinic being acquired regarding the business operations. For instance, medical safety issues and ethical standards need to be carefully assessed to avoid any discoveries of differences in professional and ethical standards:

There need to be shared values. You cannot collaborate with someone in a country far away that transfers four embryos as a standard, for example … [But] this one-embryo transfer policy, it spreads … It is the IVF model with the least [medical] complications.

(Entrepreneur, Ph.D. in Reproductive Medicine)

Third and finally, there has to be some "cultural compatibility" between the Swedish business culture and wider socio-cultural beliefs and that of the country or region wherein the new clinic is located. The entrepreneur looked to Poland, located in the Baltic Sea region to the south of Sweden and in many ways having historical bonds with Scandinavia, as one country that could be interesting to operate in. At the same time, it was not so much Poland's modern history as a communist protectorate within the Warsaw Pact under the undisputed leadership of the Soviet Union that was the concern for the Swedish firm, but the strong role of the Catholic Church, maintained throughout the Cold War era, that could be a challenge. The entrepreneur was still enthusiastic about the possibilities in Poland: "There is a certain 'Catholic issue' regarding IVF in Poland, but that is supposed to be handled now, I have been told" (Entrepreneur, Ph.D. in Reproductive Medicine).

For the IVF company, expanding the operations to e.g., Poland would broaden the basis for the operations, which in turn may help in covering the costs for e.g., advanced technologies and adding to the research budgets. The acquisition of the Polish clinics would thus enable IVF clinics to offer larger research opportunities to its co-workers. In addition, it may benefit clients if the synergies of multisite operations are exploited, leading to a larger stock of cases to learn from within the same company.

The issue of medical tourism

Regardless of the Swedish IVF companies acquiring firms abroad, there is already today a significant flow of clients that leave Sweden to seek assistance abroad. A substantial number of single women have, for instance, taken advantage of the more generous Danish policy where single women are eligible for IVF therapies. In other cases, there are couples travelling to countries where the cost is lower, e.g., the Baltic states. As Martin (2009) suggests, there are many reasons for individuals and couples seeking medical assistance abroad including national legislation, waiting times, the pricing of the therapy, or the shortage of donated reproductive material in the home market. In other words, the globalized market for reproductive medicine benefits economically favored clients and groups who can afford to travel:

Globalization makes it easier for a privileged few to cross borders in search of reproductive services or commodities unavailable or too expensive in their own countries, but it is not the great equalizer. Wealthy, elite and/or privileged consumers will have an easier time globetrotting in search of reproductive technologies than the poor and the less educated.

(Martin, 2009: 258)

One of the informants, a resident in surgery and gynecology, argued that the degree of medical tourism is quite significant and could easily be "subject to numerous Ph.D. theses." In the case of single women, the existing legislation was not widely endorsed by the clinicians even if they respected the democratic decision. The resident spoke of the present situations in terms of having "one's hands tied," i.e., the law did not leave any room for interpretation but made it clear that single women should not be catered for. However, at the same time, there was a bit of a grey zone in the case where single women could conduct gynecological examinations in Sweden while it was quite obvious that the client attempted to complete the therapy abroad. The clinicians were therefore to some extent complicit in what may be understood as a violation of the intentions of the law when they provided these health care services:

> Our hands are tied. We mustn't help these patients ... let's say I have this female patient, and she wants to be inseminated. That is not legal in Sweden, but it is legal in Denmark. She cannot just go to Denmark and announce, 'Here I am, ready for an insemination!', but that demands ultrasound analysis, an investigation. Today, that is conducted in Sweden. It is not so controversial, but in fact, it is illegal.
>
> (Resident Surgery and Gynecology,
Medical director, IVF Sweden)

This is just one of many cases indicating how legislation and "legal environments" may be quite ineffective in counteracting professional norms, beliefs, and ideologies. In the client's view, there are many good reasons for seeking assistance abroad when not eligible for the therapy in the home country, including waiting times for egg donations and age limit policies:

> Q: Why do they [clients] go abroad?
> A: Because the women need an egg donation. She cannot have that in Sweden [on short notice] ... It could be the case that she's too old – not actually *old* but old according to these 'fictive' [i.e., politically determined] age limits ... Many choose to go abroad.
>
> (Resident Surgery and Gynecology,
Medical director, IVF Sweden)

The flow of medical tourists was not only moving from Sweden to abroad, but there were also many foreign clients visiting Swedish clinics, some of the interviewees argued. A few British couples took advantage of the lower price charged by Swedish clinics, and there were couples arriving from the Middle East, possibly on the basis of the good international reputation of the Swedish clinics.

Despite this inflow of clients, interviewees by and large tended to think that it would have been better to have international standards and effective regulatory control of the clinics to reduce medical tourism. The global circulation of infertile couples and women was not something that was approved of but was treated as the effects of regional and national differences in factor prices and legislation and regulatory control.

Supplying ART to the clinics: the "outside-in view"

In addition to the clinics being the sites where IVF is conducted and where ART realized their potential, there were companies that supplied both technologies and biomedical substances (i.e., the media wherein the embryos are grown) and other resources to the clinics. As both ART and the industry mature, there are new possibilities for these categories of companies to emerge in the field. The chief commercial officer in a medical technology company, delivering a new form of incubator being equipped with a camera that enabled a more comprehensive visual history of each embryo, argued that he foresaw great market opportunities for the coming years, especially if IVF therapies would be priced at a level where it could be more widespread in new markets. The new incubator served to identify embryos that developed differently than the regular procedure:

> The [product name] is an incubator, so that's where you keep the fertilized embryos for a number of days until you implant them. In the incubator there's a constant temperature, a constant environment, so it is very safe for the embryos to develop in there. But what is special about the [incubator] is that it takes a picture of each embryo every ten minutes, so you get like a video showing you how the embryo develops. So you see the cell cleavages, you see all the special, special behavior of how the embryo develops. In the traditional clinic you take the embryo out of the incubator once a day, look at it on the microscope, so you get like one picture, and if you implant the embryo after five days you have five pictures. So now you're going to get 25,000 pictures – you get a movie. So you actually see a lot of things which you were not able to see before.
>
> (Chief Commercial Officer, Medical Technology firm)

Accessing a full visual oversight of the embryo's trajectory revealed cases where the embryo developed unexpectedly, information that informed the embryo selection work:

> Normally, an embryo will divide directly from one to two cell, to four cell, to eight cell and so on, that's the normal cleavage pattern. And, but we saw some embryos, several came directly from one to three. And maybe they will jump back to two and continue the normal cleavage pattern from there ... You immediately know that this embryo is not the best one ... We can see that some of the embryos do strange things ... And if they do these strange

things the implantation rate is much lower. So we can use all that new information to better select the most viable embryo for implantation.

(Chief Commercial Officer, Medical Technology firm)

Based on this visual information, the chief commercial officer claimed that the use of the incubator could improve the embryo selection process (measured in terms of the hard end-point data of reported pregnancies) between 20 and 40 percent, a significant figure in an industry preoccupied with performance data metrics. In addition to the analysis of individual embryos, the medical technology firm had developed a database including a large number of embryos and an algorithm that enabled the embryologists to make their choice of embryo:

Many of the customers around the world, they do upload their data so all these videos are uploaded to a central database, and we're working on that database to make what we call models or algorithms which can support in finding the most viable embryo. So the embryologist will key in the timings for each embryo, and based on these timings and these events and the embryo development the software will tell you which one is the most viable.

(Chief Commercial Officer, Medical Technology firm)

The price of the incubator was 85,000 euros, a substantial sum of money for most clinics, but since the start in 2009, there was a reported growth in demand for the incubator technology. Some clinics could choose to lease the incubator, paying per cycle and therefore getting around the high initial investment. The marketing strategy included a flat price for all clients, taking into account where in the world they were operating. This pricing policy was explained by the intense exchange of information in the field and the risk of treating clients differently. The Chief Commercial Officer explained that these contacts could extend over large geographical distances:

We have more or less the same price all over the world, because the IVF business is a very small business, and people know each other, all over the world. In my previous job I sold some incubators in Russia based on a recommendation from a embryologist in Venezuela. And I didn't know that she knew the professor in Russia. But, so you cannot just say well I have one price for you and another price for your neighbors, you need to have same price for the same type of product.

(Chief Commercial Officer, Medical Technology firm)

Moreover, the marketing was directed primarily to the clinics and not the patients, the clinics' paying customers, to avoid any unwarranted expectations regarding the qualities of the incubator:

When we're talking about branding, we are very much focused on branding not to end users but to the clinics. We try to market the product to the users of the product and not to the patients. Because it's a very sensitive area and it can very easily be misinterpreted by the patients. So, we are very reluctant in doing anything with the patient. But we would like to support our partners, in each country. With tools, with graphical events and so on, so they can do their marketing towards their customers.

(Chief Commercial Officer, Medical Technology firm)

In addition, just selling the incubator was not adding sufficiently to the firm's cash flow, so the central technology had to be combined with other product offerings and service deals. The company was therefore focused on further bundling the incubator with other resources to offer a broader set of products and services to the clinics:

Well most of [medical technology and devices suppliers] try to pull together a basket of different products for the IVF industry, based on instruments. It could be like our product, it could be like incubators or workstations. But they would also like to have some kind of consumables it could be like media, I mean where the embryos are kept during the process, or it could be plastic wear. I mean things you can sell on a regular basis, because it's difficult to build up a business only selling instruments. So, you need to have a running business of consumables as well.

(Chief Commercial Officer, Medical Technology firm)

One such product offering was a service package where the incubators were cleaned and had new filters on a regular basis, reducing the need of the clinics to be concerned about their maintenance. Also the business unit manager in a smaller biomedicine company delivering e.g., media to UVF clinics argued that it was vital to identify niches in the market to be able to compete with the major, multinational biomedicine and medical technology companies. Unless able to meet the demands of the clients and to reduce the complexity of their day-to-day work in the clinics, they would seek assistance from other competitors offering these benefits. By and large, the IVF clinics supported a growing industry of medical technology and biomedicine companies that both provided technologies and biomedical substances and tools, in turn further stabilizing and standardizing the clinical practices, leading to downward cost pressure and increased precision in e.g., embryo selection.

Summary and conclusion

When an industry has reached a certain level of maturity, standards are established and the cost-per-unit of production decreases and there are more traditional market-based activities and exchanges being established. In the case of the Swedish ART market including the IVF therapy taking place in the clinics, there are today relatively stable and predictable routines for pricing the IVF therapy through bidding procedures and cost-based pricing. As there is a high level of demand for the therapy and a good level of profit rates in the field, some of the clinics can invest in further R&D activities to both attract qualified co-workers and to develop the clinical practices. In addition, the consolidation of the field has led to at least one major private IVF company today owning six clinics and examining the possibilities of acquiring clinics abroad to further extend the cost base and to exploit synergies. Maintaining institutions thus means in practice that while there is a constant development of existing routines, there is also standard operation procedures being developed and negotiated collectively by the different actors in the field, in e.g. the complementary roles of the public and private clinics. The standard operation procedures prescribe how the day-to-day activities in the clinics should be organized, in turn setting the boundaries for the pricing of the therapies. Over time, maintenance of the institutions is needed to stabilize the field, a form of complementary work serving to accommodate the creation of new institutions discussed in the preceding chapter and the disruption of institution to be discussed in the succeeding chapter. New practices may be added to existing clinical work and incumbent ways of working may be challenged and overturned only if there is some kind of fixed point that constitutes the standard procedures.

In the general literature addressing "varieties of capitalism" (Bedu and Montalban, 2014) or "varieties of financialization" (Van der Zwan, 2014), the de-regulated market economies of the Anglo-American economies are frequently compared to the embedded liberalism and regulated economies of e.g., Germany and the Scandinavian countries, whereof the latter granting the state a more important role in developing markets and regulating relations between market actors. For scholars working in the embedded liberalism tradition, the cases of Germany, Japan, Scandinavia and other countries relying on the role of an active state are commonly treated as a curious deviation from what they tend to regard as an Anglo-American standard of the organization of the capitalist economy. In this view, e.g., the German manufacturing industry remains competitive *despite*, not *thanks to* an active state. Such an inherited view treating "unregulated markets" as being a "natural state" has a deep-rooted tradition in Anglo-American societies (Harcourt, 2011).

The turn towards market regulation and "the rolling back of the state" that began in the 1970s in the U.S. and quickly took off in the early 1980s during Ronald Reagan's presidency was in many ways a culmination of the struggle between proponents of Keynesian economic policies, granting the state a key role in stabilizing the economy, and proponents of free-market doctrines that regard the market per se as the superior mechanism for pricing commodities and optimizing the efficiency in economic transactions (Jones, 2012; Tabb, 2012; Mizruchi, 2010; Polillo and Guillén, 2005). Friedrich von Hayek, a representative of the Austrian School of Economics, was critical of John Maynard Keynes's view of the role of government in stabilizing the economy. Unlike Keynes, Hayek refused to recognize the state as a fruitful contributor to economic efficiency, suggesting that "the fundamental principle of liberalism" underlying what Hayek and his followers referred to as "economic freedom" is summarized as "the absence of state activity" (Hayek, 1949: 110). One of the principal concerns for

Hayek (1949) and other proponents of free-market capitalism is what Mancur Olson (1965) speaks of as the "free-rider problem," that the state's intervention by definition creates disturbances in what Hayek and his followers treated as self-regulating and efficient markets (Burgin, 2012). For instance, Stigler (1971) suggests that any regulation imposed by the state is designed and operated primarily "for the benefit" of the industry (Stigler, 1971: 3). In addition, when one industry receives "a grant of power from the state," the rest of the community has to bear the price for this privilege. Stigler (1971) thus proposes that regulations reduce the efficiency of the market.

This strong sense of anti-statism runs like a common thread in anti-Keynesian economic theory and policy-making, a movement including neoconservatives, neoliberals, proponents of supply-side economics, and libertarians. In this tradition of thinking, Aglietta and Rebérioux (2005: 255–256) argue, "[t]he state is perceived as a force which annihilates freedom; it is a subjugating machine." At the same time as at times quite harsh anti-statism has been articulated in both scholarly works and in popular business literature – for instance, the economist Gary Becker declared in a *Business Week* column that, "If we abolish the state, we abolish corruption" (cited in Mirowski, 2013: 220) – anti-Keynesians demonstrate a quite ambivalent view of the state as they officially and formally denounce it while in practice seek to turn it into an ally in the pursuit of economic freedom (ibid.: 56).

Outside of anti-Keynesian circles, there is a widespread belief among economic historians and economic sociologists in the role of the state as what discounts risks and provides opportunities for competitive capitalist markets. Rather than being "naturally occurring," markets are the product of skilled political action and a fabrication demanding a substantial degree of formalized laws and regulations and standards before any private equity-based initiatives to capitalize on such activities are made (Crouch, 2011: 46; Gourevitch and Shinn, 2005; Roy, 1997). Economic sociologists have argued that this skeptical view of the state, anchored in the belief in the efficiency of market transactions, is not supported by empirical evidence as states with large public sectors and active in regulating industry is in many cases capable of producing high levels of economic growth. In these two models, the neoclassical economic theory and the institutional theory model, the role of the state is regarded in entirely different perspectives; in the former, the state is a necessary evil whose influence should be minimized; in the latter, it is constitutive of the institutional and regulatory framework that embeds economic activities and economic growth.

For economic sociologists, then, the state's role is to embed and structure competitive markets wherein private venturing initiatives can be executed. "In all markets, the state is present … All markets are highly regulated. At the same time, in all markets, there is freedom," Harcourt (2011: 47–48) writes. In what at times has been described as the "neoliberal state" (e.g., Harvey, 2005: 145), the state serves the role to actively create markets where they previously did not exist (as in the case of education, health care, social security, or environmental pollution), but as soon as the conditions enabling private initiatives are in place, the state withdraws. Brown (2006: 694) suggests that rather than "facilitating the economy," in the neoliberal governance regime, the "state must construct and construe itself in market terms, as well as develop policies and promulgate a political culture that figures citizens exhaustively as rational economic actors in every sphere of life."

Especially in emerging fields or industries where the risks are high or there is a significant degree of ambiguity or uncertainty, the state must play a more active role in creating possibilities for market-based transactions (Roy, 1997). For instance, in the life sciences and in health care that involve the development of new scientific concepts and the production of new therapies and new technologies and tools, there are manifold and intricate collaborations across the private–public boundaries, in many cases in collaborative settings where e.g., research universities and start-up firms and major multinational companies exchange expertise and information in the pursuit to produce new innovations. Sunder Rajan (2012: 9) draws on the work of Jasanoff (2005) and speaks of the "co-production of life and capital" as the process wherein life is increasingly "appropriated" by capital. Sunder Rajan (2012) suggests that modern technoscience would not have been able to advance as fast as it has done unless there had been substantial economic interests in the life sciences and how economic values can be extracted from the know-how and expertise produced in both university settings and in smaller life science-based forms.

In fact, as suggested by Cooper (2008), the modern biotechnology industry is very much aligned with the liberalization and financialization of the economy beginning in the 1970s, indicating that capital supply and the investment in and the growth of the life science industry are interdependent rather than isolated processes (see also Berman, 2012: 59). Today, life science research accounts for more than 60 percent of all academic research expenditure in the U.S. (Cockburn and Stern, 2010: 3), a figure that has grown significantly since the year 2000 (ibid.: 27; Mowery, 2009: 30). In addition, the health care industry is growing and now accounts for 13 percent of the $10 trillion annual U.S. economy (Clarke et al., 2010: 57). It is important to recognize that these developments are not occurring without the state's active engagement in both funding and organizing national innovation systems and other infrastructures to benefit the development of new markets and industries.

Neoclassic economic theory treats markets as naturally occurring sites for economic transactions, an emerging field wherein supply and demand meet to price commodities at the point where these curves intersect. In contrast, economic sociologists and heterodox economic theorists regard markets as being embedded in institutional arrangements and what are shaped and informed by historical conditions and other contingencies, in many cases highly local and even idiosyncratic (Trigilia, 2002; Guillén et al., 2002; Fligstein, 2001). DiMaggio and Louch (1998) and Granovetter (1985) argue that the economy is "socially embedded," which means that economic transactions are not occurring outside of the social and cultural horizons of meaning of the market participants. This means that the neoclassical image of the market as a superior information processor, capable of apprehending and absorbing all publicly available information, is rejected as such a model represents what Granovetter (1985) speaks of as an "undersocialized theory" of the market, a site where no humans or social interests beyond the mere economic concerns are present.

In everyday conversations, markets can be referred to in such abstract terms (e.g., "the Canadian stock market" or the "global market for Brent oil"), seemingly devoid of human actors but in the everyday practices to constitute and maintain markets and market transactions there are always human beings actively involved. For instance, in the case of "risky transactions" (as in the case of IVF services, demanding much commitment from the clients), consumers are likely to use their "social ties" in their network of contacts to better predict outcomes and to reduce "opportunistic behavior" (DiMaggio and Louch, 1998: 634). In such an economic sociology view, markets are never solely constituted by calculative practices but also draw on personal contacts and other non-quantitative resources making markets not so much mechanisms for processing information and pricing commodities and services as an institutional structure wherein information and know-how is created and exchanged.

Theories about pricing what is priceless

For economic sociologists, treating markets as being socially embedded and thus contingent on local, regional, national, and international laws, regulations and other external conditions, pricing is a trickier issue than is generally recognized in neoclassical economic theory. For instance, when pricing new commodities such as electric energy, Yakubovich, Granovetter and McGuire (2005) show, there are different principles and calculative practices that can be applied, all having their own benefits and disadvantages. When it comes to the pricing of what Fourcade (2011) refers to as "peculiar goods" such as human biological tissues such as oocytes, unfertilized human eggs, the process is even further complicated. As love, children, sexuality, and a long series of basic human needs and resources that belong to the intimate sphere of the family and private life, the pricing of e.g., a child's life in the insurance industry (Zelizer, 1985) represents a "profanation" of what belong to the genera of the sacred (Zelizer, 2011: 34).

A host of research in economic sociology examines how market prices can be developed and stabilized despite social and cultural traditions rendering price-setting problematic (e.g., Fourcade, 2011; Hoeyer, 2009; Velthuis, 2007; Zelizer, 1985). Velthuis (2011: 178) studied the pricing of modern art in art galleries, not using the auction pricing mechanism but posted fixed prices for pieces of art not previously being available on the market. In Velthuis's account, the gallery owners have to carefully balance a series of objectives, traditions, and industry standards when pricing art. First of all, the formal price needs to be based on what economic sociologists call *valuation*, the inscription of social, cultural and economic value into an object. This process of valuation demands detailed expertise about the local and international art markets, the previous records of the artist, and an understanding of the present art market and economic conditions. When the object is valued, the price is set but as all modern art objects – in fact, *all* art objects – are by definition unique, the price can never be totally fixed but is based on an estimate of the demand given a series of contingencies and conditions. Velthuis explains the processes:

> Prices ... are not established by means of neutral market devices that economic agents select in order to serve their own interests, or which emerge because of their efficiency in equilibrating markets, as neoclassical economists have either implicitly or explicitly assumed. Prices are themselves embedded in the meaning structures of markets, in the preexisting institutional framework of these markets, and in the shared values of the agents who populate these markets.
>
> (Velthuis, 2011: 178)

Velthuis (2011) here speaks of *pricing scripts* as "a set of tacit, cognitive rules" which enable art dealers to "set prices systematically." These *pricing scripts* are supplemented by what Velthuis (2007: 131) names *reference values*, which "provide exact numerical values for specific pricing decisions." Velthuis' (2007) study is indicative of how prices are not only what are fixed or modified in accordance with the ups and downs of demands in e.g., spot markets, but that "prices may have many different meanings simultaneously." That is, prices are not different from other socially and culturally embedded symbols that can shift in meaning and significance (Velthuis, 2007: 170).

In the case of assisted reproduction services, the very pricing of the clinical treatment is not very complicated as it is essentially cost-based, whereof roughly 80 percent of the costs are fixed and where there is a need for each clinic or each IVF company to break even. This is attained by conducting a certain number of treatment cycles per year to secure an adequate financial performance. What complicates the pricing procedure is instead the *bidding system* that the private clinics engage in to win contracts from the regional public health care organizations that dominate the Swedish public sector health care system. As will be indicated below, the bidding system serves to pressure down the price the clients pay for the therapy in the private clinics as the present system with private and public organizations jointly enables cost-efficiency and innovation. As opposed to critics that suggest that the state is merely serving to create market imperfections, the Swedish assisted reproduction industry demonstrates a highly efficient combination of private–public collaborations that benefit the clients greatly as they can take advantage of highly advanced, state-of-the-art clinical practices at a cost that is by all standards reasonable.

7 Disrupting institutions

Expanding the legal and regulatory framework

Introduction

This third and final empirical chapter discusses how both professionals being active in the ART field, in reproductive medicine, and actors outside of the "inner circle" of biomedicine work to *disrupt* institutions and the present regime which makes it possible to open up for new activities and for new groups to advance their interests, as explained at the end of Chapter 2 in Part I of the book. The term "disruption" stresses a moment and quite violent overturning of a specific regime, but as the empirical data reported indicate, disruptive institutional work is not so much a matter of storming the Bastille as it is of participating in relatively civil and ongoing conversations and debates regarding the limits of ART and reproductive medicine. This does not suggest that there are no emotions or heated arguments involved in this work, but the inertia built into the health care and political policy-making system makes emotional outbursts quite insignificant. At the end of the day, for good and for bad, the work to disrupt institutions unfolds as a politico-administrative process concerned with the balancing of many different objectives and interests in a world of limited budgets and growing health care costs. The chapter continues by examining how actors in the field shaped the legal environment, including: the role of the legal and regulatory frameworks of practice, legal enforcement, how professionals shape the policy-making process and the sources of regulatory debates. Also, debates and critique of the legal environment and the work of patient and activist groups, with the example of gay couples advocating commercial surrogacy are further examined.

Shaping the legal environment

The role of legal and regulatory frameworks in assisted reproduction practices

The first thing to notice when it comes to the regulatory framework in the field of assisted reproduction therapies is the complex iterations between scientists and clinicians on the one hand and policy-makers and politicians on the other. Since assisted reproduction therapies are dependent on the latest advancement of new scientific know-how, the scientists and clinicians always have the upper hand as they know what is practically possible to accomplish. At the same time, they operate within a legal and regulatory framework prescribing what is permissible and what is not. "I appreciate having the regulations. They create a frame for me and for the patients. And a certain sense of predictability," one interviewee argued (Resident Surgery and Gynecology, Medical director, Private clinic). For instance, in the case of a patient seeking assistance to prepare for a planned use of surrogacy abroad, a procedure that is banned by Swedish law, the regulations leaves no room for interpretation on the part of the clinicians, the resident explained:

> If I would receive this female patient that planned for a surrogacy trip to the U.S. or something, I cannot help her. [At one occasion] I have been contacted by two companies in the U.S. that wanted me to help them with an in vitro-fertilization based on eggs procured from her ovaries. That woman was planning to use surrogacy.
>
> (Resident Surgery and Gynecology,
> Medical director, IVF Sweden)

In addition, the legal framework and the regulatory framework include international agreements and local, even regional, regulations and policies. For instance, clinically assisted reproduction is regulated by the European Union's Tissue Directive that regulates "all donation of human tissue or treatment of human tissue outside of the body" (Physiologist, Clinic #1). The physiologist claimed this was a "strict regulation," which he thought was "very good" as it clarified the rules of engagement.

By and large, the scientists and clinicians approved the strict regulation and thought it was helpful as it created legitimacy for the clinical work: "There are few other health care activities that are as monitored. Since it is a young discipline, there is much regulatory control; anything we do can be checked by someone to control how well we perform, and that is an advantage when you want things to work well," one gynecologist argued (Clinic #1). If there was any criticism articulated regarding the regulatory framework, it focused on its relative conservatism and how it limited the number of patients eligible for the therapy. The regulatory framework is "slowly liberating," one gynecologist and founder of Clinic #6 said.

One corollary of this criticism, arguably of relevance for all kinds of regulatory control, was that the regulations tended to lag behind the technoscientific and clinical possibilities and the social demands, making the regulatory framework perpetually lagging behind what is practically possible to accomplish. "I think [the regulatory framework] is outmoded. It lags behind," a resident in surgery and gynecology and the medical director of one of the major private clinics argued. "The regulatory framework is by definition lagging behind the scientific advancement in this industry," another interviewee added (Physician, CEO and Founder of Assisted reproduction clinic). One of the key concerns for the regulators is that they are trying to provide guidelines and recommendations in a field that is in a state of continuous change and modification, both in terms of what is medically and technologically possible and what the taxpayers demand from the health care system. One of the directors of the Bioethical State Advisory Board reflected on the changes over time, leading to higher expectations on the health care system:

> In 1995, this issue of IVF was not uncontroversial, this issue of having a child in an artificial way. There has undoubtedly been a change in value in society, and conventional IVF is no longer controversial ... There is also this technological development and new methods that needs to be examined.
>
> (Director #1, The Bioethical State Advisory Board)

As assisted reproduction and the use of ART have become normalized, the advancement of the biomedical technosciences leads to new issues to discuss:

> Like uterus transplantations. That was not at all on the agenda. Surrogacy was not on the agenda. Social freezing was not on the agenda. These questions regarding who owns the frozen gametes, that is, egg or sperm, was not discussed in 1995, and there are a number of additional examples.
>
> (Director #1, The Bioethical State Advisory Board)

When examining the historical development of the regulatory frameworks, one can observe that in the case of Sweden, there are two principal lines of reasoning that influence the decision-making: first, it is commonly the "rights of the unborn child" that is placed in the first room in the policy-making process. For instance, in a report issued by the Bioethical State Advisory Board on April 5, 1995 including recommendations to the Ministry of Health and Social Affairs, it is stated that, "From the state's perspective, it is of particular importance to guard the interests of the children" (Medical-Ethical Council Report, 1995: 22). This in turn translates into the proposition that "the access to assisted reproductive technologies cannot be a legal right. Such rights can only be granted if it is in the best interests of the unborn child" (Medical-Ethical Council Report, 1995: 22). Would-be parents thus hold a weaker position vis-à-vis the children born through the use of ART. Second, there has been much emphasis on what is "natural" and what "nature permits" rather than addressing practical possibilities and the expectations on the part of the clients.

In other words, much of the debate and the policy-making and legislation have been based on lines of reasoning being rooted in what may, for the lack of a better term, be common sense thinking. In some cases, the arguments are easier to understand than in others. For instance, in the 1995 report it is stated that, "The council is in agreement that egg donations to women after their menopause should be banned as it is a method that moves beyond what nature provides" (Medical-Ethical Council Report, 1995: 7). Making women beyond the age of the natural menopause undergo assisted reproduction therapies would certainly violate "what nature permits." On the other hand, in the same report, it is stated: "The council suggests that the ban on IVF including both donated egg and sperm should be continued. One of the reasons for this standpoint is that such procedures would entirely eliminate the genetic relations with the would-be parents" (Medical-Ethical Council Report, 1995: 7). In this case, the "genetic relations" – not an issue in the case of adoption – is given a priority over other social concerns including the would-be parents' willingness to give birth to a child. Later on in the report, the rationale for this recommendation is spelled out in greater detail:

> Accepting this method can be treated as a too far-reaching ambition to compensate the deficiencies of life by technical means. There is a risk that egg and sperm are handled as objects being freely available to create human beings, leading to a technological rather than a humanist view of human life. The method can be compared to embryo donation.
>
> (Medical-Ethical Council Report, 1995: 33)

As this latter argument is weaker in what virtues and values it seeks to guard and protect – the fears of a "technological" rather than a "humanist view of life" seem quite abstract as we speak of assisted reproduction and little more – and as it does not explain what undesirable effects it wants to counteract and prevent (parents caring for children conceived through the use of donated gametes are not likely to treat their children differently), the Swedish legislation today permits the use of gametes from donors. This passage in the report is complemented by the reservation of the Christian-Democratic Party director John Holmdahl, stating that "[A]ll donation of human sex cells no matter in what context should be explicitly banned" (Medical-Ethical Council Report, 1995: 70, Appendix 2). The same director also suggested that "all freezing of human embryonal individuals [sic] should be explicitly banned."

Legal enforcement

An issue that worried an interviewed politician was that recommendations and guidelines that were not fully protected by law tended to be marginalized or ignored in some of the regional public sector health care organizations. In practice, this meant that medical facts and ethical guidelines developed centrally would be subject to local interpretations when politicians are deciding what health care policies to implement. This led to a situation where there were different standards and health care services offered in different regions of Sweden, but it also tended to give unauthorized decision rights to local political bodies:

> There was a time when new methods were implemented, when the Municipality and Health Care Region Agency's [SKL, Sveriges Kommuner och Landsting] recommendation was the law. During the twelve years I have been involved with Municipality and Health Care Region Agency, in perhaps eight out of ten cases, they have been unsuccessful in advancing recommendations, both regarding fees, price-setting, or supply of therapies that are to be followed … There used to be a strict regime, almost like a

Ministry of Health and Social Affairs status, but now there is always some health care region that get an unfavourable decision and then they go home and say, 'We'll ignore that!' ... As a consequence, we advocate a stronger regime of national control regarding health care offerings and content.

(Politician, specializing in health care issues)

One of the directors of the Bioethical State Advisory Board argued that there had been long and animated discussions among the board directors whether to open up for highly regulated altruistic surrogacy in very specific cases, and added that they had reached the conclusion that surrogacy was not desirable, given the natural medical risks of any pregnancy. A key concern in the discussion about surrogacy is the concern "regarding the exploitation of females" Director #1 (the Bioethical State Advisory Board) argued. "Some say the pregnancy per se includes high risks, and that it is not acceptable for anyone to carry such risks for someone else," he continued. Still, altruistic surrogacy, Director #2 (The Bioethical State Advisory Board) admitted, "could be ethically justified to avoid any undercover commercialization." In e.g., the Netherlands, altruistic surrogacy was permitted without any economic compensation involved, and in the U.K., there was a similar legislation but with agencies serving a role in the market, one of the bioethical board members explained:

The Netherlands accepts altruistic surrogacy whereas the U.K. ... how should I put it ... rely on altruism while there are agencies coordinating ... [In The Netherlands] no money can be involved. In the U.K., there is a slippery slope caused by the presence of these agencies.

(Director #2, The Bioethical State Advisory Board)

The argument used in e.g., the U.K., that altruistic surrogacy would undermine the market for commercial surrogacy was not strong enough, nor supported by empirical evidence, the director argued; in fact, the Swedish board discussed the opposite argument, that altruistic surrogacy would serve to normalize all forms of surrogacy and therefore increase the demand. Despite these concerns, the Swedish board recognized the value of altruistic surrogacy and opened up a political debate regarding a more liberal legislation on altruistic surrogacy. In addition, there are cases of complex legal processes following gestational surrogacy arrangements, especially in cases where either the surrogate or the baby is injured during pregnancy or during the delivery:

It was claimed that there were cases in the U.K. that showed the implementation of the altruistic surrogacy policy did not lead to any fewer trips to India. And there were stories about juridical conflicts in the U.S. where the mother wanted to quit or in the case of the child as being deformed, and such things. To be honest, there are not that many such cases, but if you have been opposed to something, you always find something that speaks against the proposal.

(Director #1, The Bioethical State Advisory Board)

The two directors also argued that there were no differences between the political and regulation agency directors and the researchers and clinicians regarding the question of whether to legalize altruistic surrogacy:

> The interesting thing was that … the IVF physicians were just as unable to make up their minds regarding surrogacy as anyone else. The council shared a view, and [the medical experts] shared a view, but if you meet with a group of physicians you cannot say they are a hundred percent in agreement.
>
> (Member #1, The Bioethical State Advisory Board)

Apparently, these were complicated issues that not even detailed expertise in the clinical practices could mediate. As one of the reasons for this inability to reach a shared view is that, as one of the professors claimed, by the end of the day, altruistic surrogacy will only play a rather marginal role vis-à-vis commercial surrogacy. To some extent this was making the Bioethical State Advisory Board's work a futile attempt to counteract the growth of the global market for commercial surrogacy:

> Altruistic surrogacy, that will only play a minor role. It will not satisfy the demand. I think they calculate like 100 or 200 surrogacy births in the U.S. annually … The larger share will be commercial surrogacy, like in India and so forth for Swedish couples, I'd say.
>
> (Professor #2, reproductive medicine)

Having said that, it is not easy to have bioethical concerns and other objectives move in lockstep.

How professionals shape the policy-making process

In a field characterized by constant change and renewal, there are of necessity a number of blind spots, grey zones, and inconsistencies in the regulatory framework. For instance, while otherwise being tightly regulated, sperm donations are, "curiously enough" as one interviewee argued (Head of Clinic, Clinic #4), by and large unregulated: "Anyone can freeze sperm – you can do that! There is no law regarding for how long they can be frozen and so forth, which is quite strange considering how long you can freeze embryos" (Head of Clinic, Clinic #4). In addition, there is also a difference between the regulatory control of the clinics and the law enforcement on the level of the individual. In Sweden, single women are not eligible for assisted reproduction therapies, while in nearby Denmark they are welcome, a condition that opens up for a not negligible medical tourism to Sweden's western neighbor. This leads to a situation where single women can have their eggs retrieved and fertilized in a Danish clinic, receive the embryo, and then take advantage of full health care services in Sweden during the pregnancy despite conducting an act that is illegal by Swedish law. This is one example of how grey zones in the legal framework are a factor to consider for the clinicians:

If you're a single woman who wants a child, and there is the possibility of getting inseminated in Denmark, then you won't think 'I mustn't do this because it is prohibited by Swedish law,' but you will just go there. That is a strong driving force and will always be.

(Physician, CEO and Founder of Assisted reproduction clinic)

The case of single women being excluded from assisted reproduction therapies is one illustrative case of how the scientists and clinicians regard the regulatory framework as being "politically determined" (Gynecologist, Clinic #1) and how common sense thinking and lay beliefs influence the legal and regulatory process. In order to counteract such influences and helping to inform the policy-makers and politicians about both the opportunities and risks of novel scientific concepts and clinical practices, scientists and clinicians often take on the role of influencing the policy-making process. One of the principal arguments for such projects is that it is very complicated for non-specialists to anticipate and understand the implications of new clinical practices and their underlying science. One of the interviewees argued that it was important to inform policy-makers and politicians "just enough" so they could provide useful legislation:

We told them [politicians] just enough so they could enact the regulations … They couldn't enact regulations regarding issues they did not know was biologically possible … So all this with egg donations, embryo donations and preimplant genetic diagnostics, none of this could be predicted and anticipated … In the same manner, they were not able to foresee the freezing of embryos … We had this conflict with the authorities when we told them we stored embryos from patients with tumors being under chemotherapy and radiation therapy and at risk of losing their fertility, telling them that we won't destroy their embryos because when the patient heals they may want to get pregnant. So, we were on the verge of losing our accreditation but then they changed the law to a five years period of freezing.

(Physician and professor in reproductive medicine, Entrepreneur)

"I usually say that there are things you *can do*, things you *want to do*, and things you are *allowed to do* in a country," the interviewee continued. Not everything possible to accomplish is done, but there are still things that may be accomplished that are not yet allowed; in order to push the boundaries to accomplish things you do want to be able to accomplish, there is a need for political and regulatory action. In the following, there are a few examples of how certain issues are brought forward as pressing concerns, while some other issues are embedded in a wide-ranging consensus across the organizational field as not being subject to increased regulatory control.

Sources of regulatory debates

Standard IVF methods are today no longer controversial in the same manner they were in the 1980s or even in the 1990s, the interviewees agreed, pointing to the "normalization" of clinical practice. Still, the methodologies and techniques used in IVF therapy may be used in a variety of ways and under different circumstances, and therefore they became subject to regulatory control. In the following, some of the debates and controversies regarding legislation and policies are introduced.

PGD/PGS

As detailed in Chapter 5, the use of PGD/PGS was not an issue that could be easily resolved as medical and clinical interests and possibilities had to be weighed against ethical concerns. One of the politicians specializing in assisted reproduction policy and regulation admitted the use of PGD/PGS was controversial as there was a general concern regarding the use of know-how developed in such research work, especially among Christian groups that were visible well beyond their representation of the population in these debates:

> Lacking a background and training in health care or technological issues, certain politicians really do shudder to think about genetic diagnostics. In this country, we do actually use genetic diagnostics but in a different setting. I would not say they present a logical line of arguments, but rather adjust the message to what [policy] they want to implement.
>
> (Politician, specializing in reproductive health care issues)

As certain Christian groups were skeptical regarding assisted reproduction therapies as such, any novel concept associated with fertilization in the clinic was approached with a negative attitude regardless of its benefits and possibilities, the politician argued. Other issues that were actively debated were whether to make single women eligible for IVF therapies, and if embryos could be donated in the same way as ova and sperm could be donated. While there was not any new legislation in sight in a short-term perspective, one of the directors of the Bioethical State Advisory Board thought these issues would be handled in the coming period.

Embryo donation

The case of embryo donation was of particular interest because it would have both scientific and clinical implications. For researchers in e.g., the field of stem cell technologies, an increased supply of donated embryos would facilitate the research work. In the present regulatory regime, there is some confusion, a professor in reproductive medicine and researcher at a university hospital argued, regarding the biobank regulations. These regulations are demanding a social security number of the donor and the civil status of embryos, not being legal entities per se, and yet not fully being the "property" of the would-be parents. In this field, there was a need for a more detailed regulatory framework regarding the use of embryos after their five years in the freezer:

> We have thousands of embryos in freezers here in Sweden but we mustn't keep them longer than five years. What can we do with them after that? Is it better to throw them away than to use them in embryonal stem cell research? We believe it is better to use them. And we do have legislation permitting that with the consent of the patient.
>
> (Physician and professor in reproductive medicine, Entrepreneur)

In the clinical setting, embryo donation would enable infertile couples to receive embryos rather than just the gametes, a procedure that would facilitate pregnancies in sub-fertile couples. Clinicians approved a legal change in this respect:

> Interviewer: This issue with donating embryos?
>
> Gynecologist, Founder of Clinic #6: Well, we want that to be legalized. Right now, we keep all these frozen embryos that we will throw away after five years … You may call it an adoption. Adopting embryos is much better than adopting small children that are already born.

At present, there was no evidence of any more liberal legislation regarding embryo donation.

Age limits

Another regulatory issue that was subject to constant debate was the age limits for women in the public health sector clinics, being at different levels in the health care regions. Some of the interviewees representing the scientific and clinical community argued that the decision of what age female patients were too old for the therapy, rather than being based on robust scientific evidence regarding female fertility, was one effective means to accomplish the political objective to keep the health care budgets: "There has been some tinkering with the age limits to balance the [health care] queues, I guess. But there are different age limits in Sweden. It is quite curious that [the regulatory authorities] have been unable to determine an age limit in Sweden" (Professor #2, reproductive medicine). If the age limit is lowered, patients need to turn to the private clinics and pay for the therapies out of their own pockets, and thus public sector health care costs and queues are reduced. Also the politician being part of these decision-making processes argued that there were many lay theories circulating when these decisions were made, both on the basis of ethical and religious beliefs and financial concerns:

> In this area, I must say that there are an amazing amount of homegrown theories about delimiting the supply [of IVF therapies]. The age limits, there

we have the most restrictive and strictest rules in the country [in the Northern health care region] … I can only notice that is the case.

(Politician, specializing in reproductive health care issues)

In policy-making, advanced scientific expertise and common sense thinking are not operating in separate universes but are frequently imbricated.

Freezing time limits

The politician also argued that the maximum time period of five years for freezing gametes and embryos was another case where there was no solid scientific evidence supporting the regulatory framework. In other countries such as Finland and the U.K., this time period was extended to 10 years, a more reasonable time given the "reproductive window" of most humans in-between say the late 20s and late 30s. The politician provided an example of how the five-year rule was not very helpful for certain patients:

> This thing with freezing sperm, the one you do if you're in for some tough cancer therapy, you can only do this until you're 29. If you're 30, then 'No kids for you!' There are no private alternatives, there is nothing to do about it. Here is a series of technical rules prescribing nothing more than that we should be as restrictive as possible, for some reason.
>
> (Politician, specializing in reproductive health care issues)

Again, some policies and regulations seem to be more haphazard than grounded in scientific evidence or clinical considerations, making policy-making what is susceptible to common sense beliefs.

Debating and criticizing the legal environment

Taking action: the work of patients and activist groups to disrupt institutions

In addition to the professional groups and the regulatory and political bodies that monitor the uses of ART and IVF therapies, there are a number of patient and activist groups that work to influence the legal environment and the regulatory practices. When conducting interviews with this category of interviewees, not rooted in professional credentials or in policy-making procedures, it was apparent that there is a need for the professional community to carefully attend to the opinions and arguments articulated by these groups. While the health care organization purports to pay attention to democratic processes and to recognize emerging needs, it is still difficult to modify and change institutional settings, leading to an inertia in how e.g., health care practices are organized. At the same time, as health care deals with human well-being and human lives, this inertia is not of necessity always negatively affecting the field as there are many factors to carefully consider.

What remains clear, however, is that many patient groups believe they are being sidelined and ignored in the time-consuming and in many ways opaque procedures of issuing of reports and recommendations and policy-making occurring in the health care organization and its monitoring bodies. The chairman of a gay and lesbian rights interest organization stressed the importance of their work and pointed at the need to accumulate resources and social capital to be able to make a difference in this most difficult field of policy-making:

> We control much resources. We have our office and a clinic with 40 employees. We have a brand and a name that is well known. We have the political contacts into all parties except the Swedish Democrats [a new Right-wing populist and nationalist party]. We work well with media … We know the politicians we contact. It is not that they buy into our message, but we know what executive committees that handle different issues. We are monitoring the work in the parliament, contact the ministers and the political advisors.
>
> (National Chairman of Gay and Lesbian
> Rights Interest Organization)

Unfortunately, the chairman argued that "involuntary childlessness" was not an issue really favored by any political party for the time being. It was simply not a "privileged political issue." Despite the lukewarm interest among politicians, there were many ART issues that the organization was engaging in, not least the discrimination of e.g., lesbian couples frequently reported to the organization. First of all, the chairman argued, "there are few private clinics offering these treatments [for lesbian couples]. So the waiting time can be quite long as you are told to make use of the public sector services." Second, when being offered the therapy, lesbian couples had to pay more than heterosexual couples because they rely on sperm donations to undergo the IVF therapy. Formally speaking, the Swedish health care organization is paying allegiance to democratic virtues of equal rights, while in practice, these stated claims are hard to live up to, the chairman argued.

One case that has been frequently debated in the field, as previously mentioned, is the exclusion of single women from IVF therapies in Sweden. In July 2015, single women were made eligible for IVF therapy in Sweden, more than 30 years after the new therapy was successfully used in the country for the first time. This is not entirely flattering evidence of the inertia in policy-making in Sweden, otherwise taking pride in being at the forefront of social reforms and gender equality. For the chairman of the gay and lesbian rights interest organization, a key issue, rooted in a liberal view of individual rights, was that "people should be able to decide over their reproduction." She continued to discuss the standing concern among policy-makers, that of the child's right to have two and not just one parent(s):

> We are not opposed to the child's right to grow up with two legal parents, and so forth, but just because you don't live in a relationship that does not of

necessity mean that you don't have a broad social network. In addition, just because you have two parents, they are not always supportive and emotionally stable persons. Your childhood may not be worse just because you don't have two formal parents.

(National Chairman of Gay and Lesbian
Rights Interest Organization)

As the chairman emphasized, just making single women eligible for insemination and IVF therapies in Sweden by signing a new regulation is not enough to handle the practical problem of infertility, but the activities have to be complemented by other reforms securing the access to e.g. gametes. For this reason, the chairman praised the decision in the southernmost health care region to raise the economic compensation for egg donors from 3,000 to 11,000 crowns in an attempt to increase the activity. In addition, the organization argued that embryo donation, today banned in Sweden, would be helpful for e.g., single and lesbian women:

[The medical-ethical committee] proposed that there should be a distinction between the donation of already fertilized eggs and the donation of egg and sperm separately, but we do not share that view ... If you would introduce embryo donation, you would enable female couples with no functional ova to become parents. Today, there is no such opportunities. While other women that do not provide functional ova can become parents on basis of egg donation. Women living in partnerships with women are excluded from such opportunities.

(Chairman, Gay and Lesbian Rights Interest Organization)

In the following, the experience of two women that have chosen to be inseminated in Denmark will be discussed in order to demonstrate how this specific group of patients has had to endure a situation where their medical predicament was ignored on the basis of social norms regarding what a family in the new millennium should look like. Interviews with single mothers taking advantage of Danish IVF clinics testified to the need for taking a broader view of the infertility problem. The first interviewee started to call clinics in Sweden, in order to request help with the initial gynecological examinations to get started in the process. Already here she faced some difficulties: "I had to make phone calls to eight clinics before I found anyone willing to help me ... In one clinic, they only helped couples and unless there was a partner involved, it was 'Thank you and goodbye!'" (ART patient #1, single mother, parent of two children). In this interviewee's experience, it is an apparent act of discrimination to exclude single women from the therapy:

Once I had digested this package about being single parent and all that, I think it is discrimination to not be eligible. There is no one questioning you keeping the custody of children after a divorce, or if one parent chooses to not participate.

(ART patient #1, single mother, parent of two children)

When taking action to express her concerns regarding these political issues, representatives of political bodies responded in ways that further underlined this sense of being unfairly treated on the basis of fragile beliefs and norms:

> I have actually written two letters to [the conservative minister of social services]. The first time as an act of pure frustration over the difficulties to receive any help and wanting to inform her that was the case. The reply was that 'All children have the right to one mommy and one daddy.' I really question whether they know the legislation at all? Because lesbian couples are eligible, and in those cases there is not one mommy and one daddy.
>
> (ART patient #1, single mother, parent of two children)

Realizing that the state of Sweden would do little to help her overcome her longing for children of her own and to become a parent, the interviewee travelled to Copenhagen to take advantage of the highly developed and efficient IVF therapies being offered. Choosing a sperm donor included an "open" or "anonymous" option, with the somewhat higher price for the former. The interviewee decided to choose an anonymous donor, but could still make a choice regarding the donor's height, eye color, hair color, blood group, and level of education. In addition, the interviewee received a donation number so biological siblings could be found in the future. Being today a mother of two small girls, the interviewee was happy with her life and thankful that the insemination and the IVF therapy (in the case of the second child) worked properly. The new legislation of July 2015 was a move in the right direction, the interviewee claimed, but she did not think that it could bring the medical tourism to Denmark to a halt:

> I think there will be many traveling anyway, because there will be a shortage of donors and long waiting times, and so forth. When you go to Denmark, everything is prepared, you had these counselling conversations with them, and you can come as soon as you are ready. So, I believe many will see the benefits of handling the whole process over there.
>
> (ART patient #1, single mother, parent of two children)

The other single woman becoming a parent suffered the double stigmata of being both single and close to the age limit where IVF therapies are no longer provided, and like the first interviewee, Denmark was the destination of choice to handle the insemination problem. This interviewee thought the Swedish clinicians were very helpful despite apparently operating in a grey zone:

> My experience from Swedish doctors is that they are willing to help you. They are not so concerned about not following rules and regulations but their basic standpoint and perhaps their rationale for becoming physicians is to help people. In that case, they don't care whether you are married or not.
>
> (ART patient #2, single mother, parent of two children)

She continued:

> [Physicians] want to help, and during this process I had a number of issues I wanted to discuss with a gynecologist, so I called a private clinic in Sweden, or perhaps even several. The person answering was very kind and helpful, and said, 'These questions need to be answered by a physician but there's no physician available right now, but I can ask someone to call you up.' 'Yes, that would be fine, or I can call back later' [she replied]. 'No problem, they will call you!' After one hour, a physician calls me up, and I felt they did not have to do this because there were no formal deal that I would buy health care from them, generating any income, but they did!
>
> (ART patient #2, single mother, parent of two children)

Such stories reveal a divergence between the professional view of the present legislation and that of regulatory and political bodies, with the former group sometimes being more helpful and understanding. The second interviewee also stressed the discrimination that not only she herself but also lesbian couples encounter in the Swedish health care system:

> If a heterosexual couple seeks help, they pay the regular patient fee. But a lesbian couple would have to pay a bit more, and I assume that also a single [woman] would do so. I don't like that really, because it should be the same fee for all.
>
> (ART patient #2, single mother, parent of two children)

She continued: "Different categories of families should be treated the same way by society. That's my firm belief, but we'll see what happens next." The two single women seeking assistance in Denmark were very happy with the outcome but still deplored the inconsistencies in the Swedish legislation and health care practice, formally recognizing democratic rights while de facto acting in ways that could easily be seen as discriminating between different groups representing different sexual preferences and/or family constellation choices. Apparently there is a need for activist groups' activities to bring reproductive medicine into political debates and discussions.

Advocating surrogacy: the predicament of gay couples

The second case of activism was even more delicate to address. Single women had to fight at least two predominant ideas in the health care policy quarters, that of families being constituted by at least two adults (and prior to 2006, only heterosexual partners) and that single women are not technically speaking infertile as other IVF patients, but merely lacking the access to sperm. Yet gay men with the dream of becoming parents were for biological reasons in an even more precarious situation. Many people could easily understand and identify with women not being fortunate to find the right man with whom to have children, but it is arguably more challenging for gay men to have wider social groups accept gestational surrogacy to have their longing for children satisfied.

First, there is an element of homophobia in many societies, and while advances have been made also in Sweden, there is still, gay and lesbian groups report, evidence of discrimination of gay men and lesbians and a stable rate of so-called hate crimes in Swedish society. Also, if this group would advance the idea that their interests should be handled by more liberal legislation regarding gestational surrogacy, this causes conflict because the method is criticized by many feminist groups, otherwise often taking an affirmative view of gay and lesbian rights. In this case they are likely to receive criticism and counterarguments from feminist groups. Still, the chairman of the gay and lesbian interest organization argued that in the field of ART, new practices and technologies tended to become normalized over time, making it not entirely unthinkable that gestational surrogacy would be permitted in the future:

> What we believe to be big controversial issues today will in ten years' time be uncontroversial. I think surrogacy, being the big issue for the time being, will be treated as what is quite ordinary. If we examine this decision that same-sex couples could adopt, you notice in hindsight that the debates were totally absurd! In Sweden there is almost no adoptions made at all because of complicated legal frameworks, so in practice there were almost no children adopted by this new group.
>
> (National Chairman of Gay and Lesbian
> Rights Interest Organization)

The chairman of a pro-surrogacy organization, a gay married man and with two children born through gestational surrogacy was an ardent protagonist of gestational surrogacy. For him, it was obvious that lesbian couples' right to take advantage of IVF therapies in 2006 would open the door towards something new. At the same time, the chairman admitted, "as guys we felt a bit sidestepped, quite simply." As a response to this new situation, the chairman and a few friends started the pro-surrogacy organization, first to "serve as a hub in a network in these discussions" (Chairman, Pro-Surrogacy Organization) and to provide a home page and a forum for exchange of ideas, as well as where journalists and researchers could contact individuals who are engaged in the issue.

Eventually, the number of participants and interested individuals grew in number and the organization received some media attention. Having experience from gestational surrogacy himself, the chairman had been invited to tell his "story" a number of times to journalists who were eager to address this most heated topic. Both his children, a four-year-old girl born at the time of the interview and a boy born in 2013, had been born in India and involved, as he said, four women: "Two egg donors and two surrogate mothers."

The chairman argued that the attention from media and from policy-makers has grown over the years, and ten years ago, around 2003–2004, "this was a question that flew under the radar, you could say," the chairman claimed. The early work of the interest group included the ambitious project to read all "government reports" and so forth to figure out what they stated and assumed regarding gestational surrogacy. As the chairman argued, the official view of surrogacy was burdened by an unwillingness to address the issue at all: "It was a bit like in the case of zoophilia in old legal texts, where there is this avoidance of the term altogether, so people don't get the wrong idea" (Chairman, Pro-Surrogacy Organization). In his reading of some of the documents, one of the reasons for treating surrogacy with utmost skepticism was that it was at an early stage realized that it would be of interest for the gay community in the case of a more liberal policy regarding IVF:

> During this investigation regarding lesbians being eligible for insemination, they sent out this report for commenting to the regional health care organizations ... I believe it was the Västra Götaland Region that responded, 'Well, we do think this sounds reasonable for this group. But if we make this group eligible, then the male gay community will instantly advance their right to surrogacy. In other words, we are not supporting this proposal.'
> (Chairman, Pro-Surrogacy Organization)

Treating such a declaration as being part of a long-standing tradition of anti-gay policies and cultural rejection of gays and lesbians, the chairman argued that there was evidence of quite alarming formulations in this body of formal documents:

> The State of Sweden's Medical-Ethical Council, they thought surrogacy was so appalling that children born this way would reasonably wish they were not born this way ... They wrote: 'From the child's perspective, it cannot be considered desirable to be born under these conditions.' That is possibly the cruelest formulation I have seen in my entire life! There are physicians and people working with these issues, using their authority to make the claim that if you are born through surrogacy, you should wish you were never born at all!
> (Chairman, Pro-Surrogacy Organization)

Over the years, the chairman had experience from numerous debates, panels, televised discussions, and so forth, and he firmly believed there are few, if any, arguments against surrogacy that are not based on inherited folk beliefs regarding either family life per se or gay men:

> I believe I am well informed when it comes to debates and so forth. Over the years, I have been yearning for a proper contestant presenting adequate arguments, but all I encounter are these emotional arguments, 'This ain't no good!' 'But please tell me why this is not good?' 'Well, I just feel this ain't no good!' 'Well, fine, but on what do you base this judgment?' [Laughter].
> (Chairman, Pro-Surrogacy Organization)

There are, the chairman argued, many home-grown theories about mothering and parenting that are mobilized to maintain the ban on surrogacy, for instance the idea that the mother and the child create a special bond during the pregnancy, an idea that the chairman claimed was more based on a romantic and gendered idea about mothers than based on solid empirical evidence. A more pressing concern was the critique that surrogacy represents a commodification of the female reproductive capacities and in particular when surrogacy arrangements are made in poor countries where uneducated women serve the role as the surrogates. The chairman understood and was very familiar with that claim, but responded that his experience was that it was equally unjust that middle-class women with an interest in feminist issues would serve as self-declared spokesmen of these women. Instead, he argued, these women were "upset when they learn that there are women [in the West] who speak on their behalf," denying them the right to earn the money from giving birth to a baby:

> These women say, 'It is not their thing to decide whether we want to be here or not!' It is very, very interesting that women being self-declared feminists and taking a firm pro-choice position, that they do not allow other women to make their own choices. It is like they oppose their integrity when it comes to this issue … I regard that as being patronizing and as an arrogant attitude, and that is quite daunting.

> (Chairman, Pro-Surrogacy Organization)

As gay men and women may, at least in theory, share the sense of being marginalized or serving as the Other to the white, middle-class male, the critique from feminists regarding the economic inequality that lies at the heart of the surrogacy arrangement is too complicated to ignore. In response to this criticism, the chairman argued that the Indian women were recruited from the "lower middle class or upper working class" and that all of them have been through pregnancies previously, indicating that they know very well what to expect. In e.g., the U.S., he continued, surrogates tend to be "deeply religious women," treating their work as the "ultimate gift, quite simply" (Chairman, Pro-Surrogacy Organization). While the chairman argued that it would cost roughly one million Swedish crowns to engage an American surrogate mother including all expenses, the total cost in India would be perhaps one fourth of that amount of money. In the U.S., the process was more like a form of "dating process" where it is the surrogate mother that choses which persons she wants to help. In contrast, he added, based on his own experience of India, "things are more 'industrialized,' to put it like that" (Chairman, Pro-Surrogacy Organization).

Both the chairman of the gay and lesbian interest organization and that of the pro-surrogacy organization shared the belief that as time proceeds, there will be new attitudes and changes that are hard to predict and anticipate from today's perspective. If time worked in their interest, the more short-term issue was how to speak at all about surrogacy without violating too many inherited beliefs and social norms. The chairman of the pro-surrogacy organization explained that one of the members of the parliament had addressed the term surrogacy itself, having the connotation of artifice and "being associated with surrogate products used during the war." Instead the term "host mothers" was suggested, but the chairman was not so enthusiastic about this idea: "For our generation, that makes us think of *Alien* [Ridley Scott's science-fiction/horror movie (1979)]" (Chairman, Pro-Surrogacy Organization). The chairman of the gay and lesbian interest organization also claimed that it was not really helpful to speak about parenting as some "natural right." She preferred to reason on the basis of what is technically and socially possible to accomplish at present:

> We do not debate the surrogacy question as a kind of civil rights issue, or an anti-discrimination issue or anything similar. We need to stress that position. We need to be quite specific regarding parenting not being 'a natural right' or so, for instance. But we are concerned about discrimination in legal texts, as in the case where female couples were excluded from assisted conception therapies ... It would look odd to claim that it is a case of discrimination when there are no possibilities for the legal right to use surrogacy. That would be a peculiar form of rhetoric.
>
> (Chairman, Gay and Lesbian Interest Organization)

The chairman of the gay and lesbian interest organization also agreed with her colleague that there were many ideas being articulated without being thoroughly grounded in any solid evidence: "The Female Physicians' Organization have declared a ban on surrogacy, but I really do not know why that is the case, but they are quite alone in making this statement, right!" Moreover, the chairman argued, based on a medical journal article, that it is curious that uterus transplantation is permitted, as a much more medically complicated and uncertain way to promote human fertility than surrogacy, while surrogacy is banned.

Regardless of the overtly skeptical view among policy-makers and the wider public, the chairman of the pro-surrogacy organization claimed that he was every now and then contacted by women that declared their ambition to become surrogate mothers and inquired where to turn. Still, the question of commercial gestational surrogacy seemed very much shaped by the concern for the exploitation of (especially) poorer women, and not so much that surrogacy is "unnatural," a condition that perhaps underscores the normalization and familiarization of the IVF therapy. Retrieving eggs, fertilizing them with donated sperm, and transferring the embryo to a third person's womb was per se not treated as a conspicuous violation of nature but was instead widely understood as a staple method for producing pregnancies. The crux with surrogacy is just that not only the egg and the sperm are paid for but that also the uterus is now subject to pricing negotiations.

All the activists doing their best to modify the existing system both to help themselves become parents and to make things easier for the coming generation, hopefully better recognized as legitimate users of ART without the need to fight their corner to become eligible for the therapy. As one of the single mothers aptly summarized that at the end of the day what matters here and now is individual accomplishment, and not dry policy-making activities: "I am happy with how my life has become, and I intend to continue to be happy, regardless of how the legislation develops" (ART patient #1, single mother, parent of two children).

Summary and conclusions

The regulatory limits of professional practices

At the heart of biomedical technosciences is the drive to constantly develop new, more effective, and safer practices, and therefore the legal and regulatory framework tends to be "pulled" by scientific breakthroughs rather than the legal and regulatory framework "pushing" policies and recommendations into scientific communities. In addition to biomedical technosciences, social changes and new attitudes towards family life and parenting create additional pressure on legislators and regulatory bodies. The Swedish legislation, excluding single women from taking advantage of assisted reproduction therapies, was thus at risk of being outmoded and out of step with social norms and the social realities of women no longer of necessity demanding conventional family structure to create families.

Second, regardless of the legislation and regulatory frameworks, the causes of this inertia may have been *social concerns* as in the case of Sweden where the legislation very much emphasizes the rights of the unborn baby, *ethical norms* regarding e.g., the risks of an expanded use of genomics methods when selecting embryos for transfer as in the case of the use of PGD/PGS, and *religious beliefs* regarding e.g., the legitimacy of reproductive medicine at large or the legal status of lesbian couples. Third, legislation and regulatory framework are never conclusive and prescribing practices in every detail, but there is always room for professional judgment and evaluation, and there are always omissions, grey zones, inconsistencies, and possibilities for interpretations in any regulatory framework. Scientists and clinicians are also partners in creating the legal and regulatory frameworks, but their vested interests are counterweighted by the presence of laymen (often politicians or patient group representatives) in e.g., the ethical committees and advisory boards that issue reports and recommendations to legislative bodies. That is, "informational asymmetries" benefitting the scientific and clinical community are handled by increased representation of non-expert groups.

Fourth and finally, in certain cases, legal and regulatory framework may in fact lack standards and widely recognized calculative practices which enables the effective implementation and enforcement of a law or regulation (Lakoff and Klinenberg, 2010). This lack of standards opens up for "politics" and "negotiation" and therefore renders the legislation inefficient. In other words, the relationship between legal and regulatory frameworks and organizational practices demonstrates what may be referred to as "garbage-can like qualities" (after the garbage-can theory of organizational decision making, see Cohen, March, and Olsen, 1972; March and Olsen, 1976). In other words legal and regulatory frameworks and organizational practices are not always connected in a linear and sequential manner as novel practices may create new regulations in the same way as new regulations caused by e.g., new international standards may influence a practice.

Common sense thinking may render such legal and regulatory "flexibilities" and "dynamics" as evidence of a faulty articulation allowing loopholes and grey zones. Still, if the role of law is to be seen, as legal scholars propose, as a "neutral medium" that offers "a universal means through which anyone can negotiate with anyone" (Gershon, 2011: 541), such interpretative spaces must be tolerated. For example, laws serve their functions best when they define entities (e.g., participants in a market) as equal, or at least commensurate, "despite wide disparities in size and internal organization" (ibid.: 540). To take on this image of being neutral and capable of safeguarding everyone's autonomy, laws need to be *general*; they must be constituted by written legal texts but also accompanied by skilled interpretations and enforcement. This is true not the least in the domain of health care practices, being constantly riddled by ethical concerns and difficult decisions, and consequently there are numerous ethical committees and boards monitoring health care organizations.

In order to "disrupt institutions," to render them de-familiarized and no longer taken for granted, potentially even being a source of healthy suspicion, the agent engaging in this work needs resources. The legitimacy of the claims made in the attempt to disrupt institutions can either derive from expertise or a central and authoritative location in a field, or be based on moral claims. Facts and figures are the principal outcome from scientific investigations and procedures, but the moral authority of such data must always, in a democratic and open society, be determined by wider social communities including non-experts. In the case of these non-experts being sidelined, the governance of a field deteriorates to mere technocracy, and from history we may learn that it is in the long-term perspective an undesirable scenario (see e.g., Péteri, 1989). The legislative and regulatory activities that serve to stabilize institutions and to discount risks and balance the interests of various stakeholders must always be able to adapt to novel research findings, clinical practices and innovations, as well as to ideas and beliefs that are articulated outside of expert communities.

In this view, there are at least three social resources that are included in the institutional work to disrupt institutions. First, there is professional expertise and practices, the totality of activities endorsed and conducted by professional groups within a field. Second, there is what may be referred to as the *moral economy* of the field, the professional practices embedded in widely shared social norms and beliefs regarding what are legitimate professional practices. This concept will be examined in more detail shortly. Third, there is a legal environment (Edelman, 1990) constituted by legal and regulatory frameworks that bridge and co-align professional practices in a specific field and the wider social norms and beliefs. The legal environment commonly rely on expertise of relevant professional groups, but must at the same time pay attention to lay beliefs in order to not distance the legislation from everyday norms. Technocratic governance is characterized by the willful ignorance of lay beliefs and legislators should therefore ensure that there are mechanisms in place that can accommodate what non-expert communities also want to accomplish.

The concept of moral economy is a key term in e.g., economic sociology, suggesting that e.g., legislation and juridical contracts cannot operate and be enforced unless there are implicit assumptions made regarding the obligations of the contracting parts. That is, "the economy" as an abstract system of monetary exchanges and the circulation of goods and services cannot operate without a foundational and shared (at least by the majority) moral belief. "By *moral economy* I mean a system of transactions which are defined as socially desirable (i.e., moral), because through them social ties are recognized, and balanced social relationships are maintained," Cheal (1988: 15) writes. As Daston (1995: 4) remarks, the term "moral" carries connotations to eighteenth- and nineteenth-century moralism, a stern and patriarchal view of where the line of demarcation between what is right and what is wrong is to be drawn, but in the concept of moral economy, the term moral refer to both psychological and normative elements regarding what is legitimate social action. This economic sociology view of the moral economy leaves us with institutional work aimed at disrupting institutions as being what is balancing between the ability to advocate either new professional expertise or to address issues that are rooted in a communal belief that the existing institutional order is not sufficiently balancing interest and/or exploiting the full potential of a specific resource.

The role of laws and regulations in shaping markets

In the general tendency to liberalize and de-regulate markets and economies after 1980, there has been a widespread belief in laws and regulations as what imposes unnecessary complications on what are treated as self-regulating markets. What at times have been referred to as neoliberalism or free-market liberalism is a wide policy and intellectual movement away from state regulation (Tomaskovic-Devey and Lin, 2011: 556), based on the assumptions that markets work best when they are left on their own. In what at times are called *liberal market economies* of the Anglo-American model of the U.S. and the U.K. (Bedu and Montalban, 2014: 38), there has been a firmer belief in the virtues and efficiency of deregulation, at times leading to disastrous outcomes as in the case of the 2008 finance industry collapse. The finance crisis that was, Princeton economist Alan Blinder (2013: 344–345) argues, "the result of a series of grievous errors, misjudgments, and even frauds by *private* companies and individuals, aided and abetted by a hands off policy from a government unduly enarmored of laissez-faire." "America was plainly a victim of *too little* regulation, not *too much*," Blinder (2013) adds (see also Friedman and Kraus, 2012; Stiglitz, 2010).

In contrast, a large number of organization theorists, science and technology researchers, and legal scholars demonstrate that robust legal and regulatory frameworks serve to stabilize and standardize emerging professional and technological fields and to create possibilities for economic growth (Gourevitch and Shinn, 2005; Roe, 2003; Roy, 1997). "Regulation generates results, raises questions and produces phenomena whose significance feeds into the practices that are the subject of regulatory activities," Cambrosio et al. (2006: 195) claim, and point at the role of the state and international bodies as legislators and regulators, especially in emerging fields or markets (Bozanic, Dirsmith, and Huddart, 2012; Abdelal, 2007; Singer, 2007; Vogel, 1996). In addition, in many cases, there is evidence of iterative processes wherein regulation and innovations are not unidirectional but where, Abraham and Reed (2002: 338) write, "scientific and technological innovations can influence regulatory developments." Such iterative loops where regulations and innovation practices are mutually adjusted may be effective in promoting novel products and services, but there is always a risk of either participant advancing its own agenda or gaining an upper hand over other participants (Hiatt and Park, 2013; Abraham and Davis, 2009).

The legal environment

What Edelman (1990) refers to as the legal environment, envisages laws and regulations as: (1) being general and always open for some local interpretation; (2) demonstrating what Merton (1936) called "unintended consequences of purposeful action." Institutional theory, "old" (Selznick, 1949) as well as "new" (Meyer and Rowan, 1977), regard organizations as social systems that are open to external influences and that are contingent on its environment. In order to secure long-term survival, organizations must therefore constantly adapt to and modify to accommodate these external pressures and changes. At the same time, organizations need to protect their core activities from such influences and in many cases this is accomplished through a decoupling between actual activities in the core and the symbolism and rhetoric at the periphery of the organization (Thompson, 1967). It is useful to theoretically distinguish, as Fligstein (1996: 658) does, between *institutions* as being the "shared rules, which can be laws or collective understandings, held in place by custom, explicit agreement, or tacit agreement," and *governance structure*, which refers to "the general rules in a society that define relations of competition, cooperation, and market-specific definitions of how firms should be organized." Laws and regulatory framework are commonly regarded as what bridge institutions and governance structure as they both prescribe *how* organizations should act in certain fields at the same time as these laws and regulatory frameworks influence and shape competition and collaborative activities in industry. In the ideal case, laws and regulations are thus both setting the limits for market activities and serve as a vehicle for improved efficiency (e.g., Faulkner, 2012).

In this general analytical framework, laws and regulations are part of the organization's environment, a set of legal, regulatory, and normative rules and principles that need to be followed and adhered to (Stryker, 2003). At the same time, these rules and principles are at times not enforced without substantial costs, and therefore there is some leeway in how organizations implement routines and standard operation procedures to accommodate legal frameworks. This does not suggest that organizations act opportunistically, and there is evidence of legislation that is relatively vague being translated into quite ambitious organizational change programs, including the growth of professional human resource management departments in e.g., American industry (Baron, Dobbin, and Jennings, 1986; Sutton et al., 1994), organizational responses to anti-trust laws (Dobbin and Dowd, 2000), or to civil rights legislation (Kelly and Dobbin, 1999). The development of such practices and new organizational units signal the organizations' "commitment to compliance" to handle federal regulations, despite a lack of exact prescriptions on how to act (Dobbin and Sutton, 1998).

In the work to discount risks and institutionalize standard operating procedures for market exchanges, laws and regulations play a decisive role. Institutional theory scholars, science and technology researchers, and legal scholars have emphasized how laws and regulations structure a variety of activities including corporate governance (Fligstein and Choo, 2005), shareholder value creation (Stout, 2013, 2012; Rock, 2013; Bratton and Wachter, 2010), the creation of innovations and new markets (Faulkner, 2012; Ashford, Ayers, and Stone, 1985), clinical practices (Pickersgill, 2012), and in creating intellectual property rights, widely recognized as what shapes innovative industries (Pottage, 2011; Sell, 2003). Studies of legal and regulatory control have also revealed how finance market trading (Bozanic, Dirsmith, and Huddart, 2012) and finance market rating practices (Partnoy, 1999) are informed by regulatory frameworks and their enforcement. In the field of assisted reproduction and clinical practices, several scholars have examined the effects of lack of international agreement in e.g., commercial gestational surrogacy (Mohapatra, 2012; Smerdon, 2008), and how legal frameworks that purport to balance the interest of a variety of stakeholders are blind to e.g., race and class issues (Leong, 2013).

These studies show that law and regulation constitute a *legal environment* wherein laws have important *indirect effects* on organizations, i.e., laws and regulations are not enacted in the pursuit of the highest possible efficiency and control in organizational governance but seek to create a regulatory framework that *guides* rather than *prescribes* organizational action and managerial practices (Edelman, 1990: 1402–1403).

As a consequence, as opposed to the neoclassical economic theory view of market regulation, privileging *efficiency* over *stability*, legal scholars justify the wider legal view wherein many different interests and objectives need to be effectively balanced: "The corporation was after all a delegation of sovereign powers to serve the public interest, thus the corporation did not grow by an evolutionary process by which an organizational form was perfected to its maximum efficiency," Roy (1997: 76) writes as a response to critics of corporate law as being an unnecessary complication, inhibiting the realization of full market efficiency. Instead, as Edelman (1990: 1436) shows, new laws may in some cases lead to organizational changes being greater – and different – from what was intended by lawmakers; legal and regulatory frameworks never fully determine organizational practices.

The literature on legal and regulatory control of corporations and industries thus suggests that laws do play a central role in shaping managerial practices of industries. At the same time, Edelman, Fuller, and Mara-Drita (2001: 1595) suggest that the law is "broad and ambiguous and is rarely read directly by employers." Instead, employers rely on legal consultants that interpret and filter the law "through a variety of lenses," leading to a "managerialization of law," the process by which conceptions of law may become (with a term first used by Selznick [1949]), "[p]rogressively infused with managerial values as legal ideas move into managerial and organizational arenas" (Edelman, Fuller, and Mara-Drita, 2001: 1592). In this account, this infusion of "managerial values" into law may reframe the law in ways that "make it appear more consistent with traditional managerial prerogatives" (ibid.). That is, unlike the free market capitalism argument, resting on the efficient market hypothesis suggesting that the market is a superior mechanism for economic transactions as market actors jointly accommodate publicly available information in the ongoing and ceaseless process of pricing, scholars examining legal and regulatory frameworks suggest that law is not of necessity a regressive force to consider but may also establish the standards and routines needed to advance new innovation, industries, and markets. In other words, as suggested by Halliday and Carruthers (2007), there is a *recursivity* between law and managerial action and organizational practice – law and managerial practices shape and inform one another.

Seen in this legal environment perspective, this study contributes to the institutional theory literature that examines the connections between legal frameworks and organizational practices (e.g., Zorn, 2004) and structures (e.g., Baron, Dobbin, and Jennings, 1986). One important contribution from this literature is that while, as Edelman (1990: 1402) writes, "law creates, and helps to constitute, a normative environment to which organizations must adapt." It is worthwhile to note again that the relationship between law and organizational practice is not always unidirectional; in some cases, e.g., a new regulation may affect the organizational practice (Cambrioso et al., 2006: 195); in other cases, as Abraham and Reed (2002) detail in the case of antidepressant drug development standards (see also Lakoff, 2012, 2007; McGoey, 2010), preferable and widely established practices may in fact serve to influence the regulations.

Part III
Institutionalizing ART

8 The making of
reproductive futures

Introduction

As philosophers of technology and students of science and technology have emphasized time and again, both science and technology are man-made creations that in their own idiosyncratic ways make their claims on the future. The basic idea of science and technology – technoscience – is to enable a better future for human beings and for coming generations. But this narrative to already here and now colonialize parts of the future – as Louis Althusset reminded us, the future lasts a long time – is curiously vague in what these promises and expectations actually mean. This is in part due to the opaque term of the future per se as "time that will come," in part caused by the imprecision of such statements, as being more based on hopes and wishful thinking than an actual ability to anticipate futures. While the present and the past may be confusing and contained in ambiguities, beset by controversies regarding how to write history and how to govern the present period, the future is always of necessity uncertain and open for expectations. Yet, it is this uncertainty that is appealing for human beings, for politicians, scientists, visionaries, but also prophets and doomsayers predicting calamities around the bend. In short, the future is deeply intriguing for humans. In addition, as Blaise Pascal noted, it is the future and the future only that is our destination, and perhaps increasingly so in the high-paced society of late modernity:

> We almost never think of the present, and if we think of it, it is only to see what light it throws on our plans of the future. The present is never our end. The past and the present are our means, the future alone our end. Thus we never actually live, but hope to live, and once we are always planning how to be happy, it is inevitable that we should never be so.
>
> (Pascal, 1966: §67, p. 13)

Human lives are indeed, as St. Augustine put it, cast in "the long shadow of the future." Such existential predicaments can however be used purposefully by e.g., proponents of technologies and scientific programs; colonializing bits and pieces of the future to advance their own interest and render their commitments legitimate.

Selin (2007), speaking about nanotechnology, a primary example of such colonialist tendencies in the technosciences, stresses how the future is always already discounted in the nanotechnology discourse:

> Technologies are not merely tools that are used or applications of science that are discovered, but rather are made through claims and counterclaims and constructed in one way rather than another, which is stabilized in social and material structures.
>
> (Selin, 2007: 199)

Speaking about nanotechnology, Selin (2007: 197) proposes, technoscience includes a "colonializing the future." Milburn (2004: 123) shares this view, extending the argument to say that the nanotechnology discourse from the very beginning advanced a form of hybrid narrative, "punctuating the fragile membrane between real and simulation, science and science fiction, organism and machine, and heralding metamorphic futures and cyborganic discontinuities." In advancing this new view of the possibilities of technology at the nanoscale, the present regime of humanism is criticized from the "vantage point of an already inevitable future" (ibid.).

While nanotechnology is one of the areas of scientific expertise yet to prove its social value to fulfill these grandiose plans for mankind, this colonialization of the future has occurred at many historical points. For instance, Nye's (1990: 66) analysis of the electrification of the major North American and European metropolises was based on the idea of a "brilliant future for civilization." The popular press saw in the new electric light a "white magic" that foreboded an "electrical millennium" (ibid.). In this view, scientists, engineers, and others developing new technoscientific contributions are engaging in what Fine (2007: 102) – studying meteorologists – calls "futurework." The future is yet to come, but already at this point of time, at the tipping point of the future, the proponents of technosciences make claims to know what can happen, or better, what can be made to happen. Abraham Lincoln famously declared that "The best way to predict the future is to create it," and no social group has remained more faithful to this proposition than proponents of the technosciences.

The crux is just that while visionaries may be fully convinced about their land-marking accomplishments, the surrounding society may be less animated by such hopes for the future but may be mildly interested in e.g., "nanofutures" or even be hostile to the indecency of trying to accomplish novel technologies and scientific procedures. Many entrepreneurs have been forced to bite the dust when recalcitrant populations have refused to recognize their contributions. Stability and change move in lockstep in human societies and advanced capitalist economies, and frequently what Joseph Schumpeter spoke of as the "entrepreneurial spirit" is precisely this understanding of "when the time has come" for a particular idea. Entrepreneurship is thus not only engaged in the creation of new ideas and concepts, but also with the social activities that make these ideas viable and recognized outside of the more narrow circles of experts.

In the final chapter of this volume, the empirical material reported in Part II of the book will be examined in terms of its contribution to organization theory and management studies, to the study of ART and reproductive medicine, and to policy-making. Reproductive medicine and its clinical application has been thoroughly grounded in the belief that the future is man-made and that human intelligence can be mobilized to handle issues and concerns that are seemingly insurmountable. Like many other technoscientific fields, there is a pantheon of researchers, clinicians, activists, and policy-makers that have jointly contributed to the present situation where sub and infertile couples and single women no longer had to put their hopes to prayers but where advanced state-of-the-art medical research expertise can help them become parents. But as humans and as researchers and clinicians, the future alone is our end, and therefore there is ongoing and ceaseless work to make therapies better, safer, and less painful. In short, these humans engage in making the reproductive future of mankind.

The three forms of institutional work

Based on the review of the institutional theory literature in Chapter 3 of this volume, the three ideal-typical forms of institutional work of Lawrence, Suddaby and Leca (2009) was used to structure the empirical material collected in the study of ART and reproductive medicine. First, the advancement of social freezing as a clinical practice and commercial service offering, the extended yet highly regulated and controlled use of PGD/PGS, and the more visionary and future-oriented research work to transplant wombs into female bodies to help them become mothers, were three cases that shared the ambition to create new products and services. The long-term consequence of this work was to create new institutions including not only clinical practices and laboratory routines but also novel social beliefs, norms, and identities. Second, institutional work that maintains institutions include a variety of practices that tend to be less conspicuous than the creation and disrupting of institutions. In this setting, maintaining institutions means negotiating and establishing routines for how the clinics can price their therapies and services and how they can balance the need for financial stability and transparency and long-term commitment to R&D and other developments. The pricing of therapies demands standard and regulatory frameworks so relevant actors can learn on what basis they will be evaluated and how to be competitive within such standardized frameworks. In the case of ART, the institutional work to maintain institutions is very much a matter of private companies handling their day-to-day businesses. In the field of IVF therapies, regulatory agencies and the state have today discounted many of the risks and therefore there are good opportunities for privately owned companies to supply the bulk of the clinical practices.

Third and finally, the institutional work to disrupt institutions is less the work of professionals and insiders as in the case of institution creation or the work of company representatives as in the maintenance work, operating on the basis of widely accepted routines for the governance and managerial control of private enterprises and public clinics. Disruptive institutional work is instead likely to emerge in the margins of the institutional and organizational field when e.g., interest groups, clients, patients, and other non-professional stakeholders engage in the work to shift the focus on how the field is organized. At the same time as these groups may have relatively limited influence on e.g., legislative and regulatory practices, as they are outsiders, the legal environment of a particular field and its regulatory control must be capable of responding and adapting to new social beliefs and expectations. Many interviewees argued that IVF practices were initially met with great skepticism in the 1980s and there were many dismissive comments about "test-tube babies" and "baby-factories," but that this attitude has been successfully overcome by the sheer success of the IVF therapy per se.

As these new reproductive possibilities have been recognized, new demands surface. In some cases, the predominant health care policies and political decisions are not based on medical considerations. Often policies are, however, rooted in norms and beliefs regarding family structures and e.g., lesbian women and single women have historically been treated as individuals failing to meet such baseline standards. In these cases, policies can quite easily be changed through modifications in existing legal and regulatory frameworks. In other cases, most noteworthy the case of gestational surrogacy advocated by some interest groups, the medical and clinical practices do not need to be modified but rather include more individuals (e.g., would-be parents, egg donors, surrogates). Such an arrangement is seated in social, cultural, and not the least juridical complexities that may be too complicated to practically handle.

While gay men argue that their best bet to become parents would be commercial gestational surrogacy, this claim needs to be understood against the debate regarding the ethics of paying for gestational surrogacy, including the concern that pregnancies always of necessity include biological risks for both the surrogate and the baby. While some groups argue that gestational surrogacy is by definition a deplorable commodification of female reproductive capacities and therefore violates norms about human dignity, "what nature allows," and similar vague but yet culturally embedded beliefs, others tend to point at the juridical difficulties involved in designing the contracts between the parts. Under all conditions, the work of this interest group operates outside of the core of the institutional field and encounters a series of difficulties in accomplishing a wider recognition of their interests. Despite all this resistance to surrogacy, the Medical-Ethical Board has today opened up for an extended discussion on the possibilities for altruistic surrogacy in certain cases, a shift in their policy-making that suggests that future generations may regard surrogacy differently.

All vital institutional and organizational fields include these three forms of institutional work. As in the case of ART in Sweden, without the creation of institutions, the field stagnates and fails to attract creative and innovative individuals who can further develop the existing practices. When it comes to institutional maintenance work, the maturing field needs to establish standards for how to calculate and price products and services to be able to reduce the cost per treatment cycle. This is the day-to-day management of the activities of the field.

Finally, without at least the potential risk of the existing institutional field being questioned and problematized from "the fringes," the professionals operating in the core and regulating the field may fail to respond to societal changes and novel social demands and expectations. Various stakeholders' claim the right to take advantage of e.g., clinical practices and therapies is ultimately the evidence of the attractiveness of the services offered. But as e.g., professionals and certain interest groups (say gynecologists and single women) may share the belief in the importance of providing the therapy to new groups, there are regulatory and political bodies monitoring the field that also have the mandate to influence the decision. The capacity to keep all these activities in balance through these three forms of institutional work are what makes a field vital and responsive to social changes.

The role of ART and reproductive medicine in contemporary society can be summarized in Table 7.1 below.

Table 7.1 The three forms of institutional work

	Creating institutions	*Maintaining institutions*	*Disrupting institutions*
Focus	Scientific development	Economic conditions and enterprising activities	Legal, regulatory, and normative changes
Key actors	Scientists in reproductive medicine, clinicians	Managers, clinicians	Political bodies, ethical committees, activist groups
Actors' position in the field	Central	Intermediary	Peripheral
Principal outcomes	New ART possibilities	The market-making and pricing of ART offerings	The legal and regulatory control of clinical practices and market-based activities
Key sources of knowledge and expertise	Scientific, clinical	Managerial skills, calculative practices, and marketing know-how	Political skills, policy-making competence, activist work

Contribution to organization theory and management studies

The study of ART and reproductive medicine adds to the organization theory and management studies literature a case of how institutional fields are constituted through the three processes of institutional work. Much institutional theory, the "classic" as well as the neo-institutional theory view, is preoccupied with stability and the transfer of practices, standards, and organizational forms between institutional fields and industries, making change, if not exceptional, at least a matter of imitation of what already exists elsewhere in e.g., adjacent fields or professions. The three forms of isomorphism examined by DiMaggio and Powell (1983) is exemplary of how change is treated as being based on various forms of adoption of existing practices and organizational forms. In contrast, more recent contributions to institutional theory literature have been more concerned about the question of change and novelty, making the question of agency a key theoretical concern.

In the recent literature, agents can act as "entrepreneurs" within institutional fields, or different "institutional logics" serve to animate actors to behave in accordance with certain norms and beliefs. In these two views, the actor is suddenly inscribed with certain enterprising capacities, or they remain more or less under the influence of predominant institutional beliefs, but still are capable of acting freely within these confines. Institutional work is instead based on the idea that actors are infused with agency but that their work is structured on the basis of an institutional framework, making the agent neither a freely enterprising individual, nor a "cultural dupe" only capable of thinking and acting in accordance with instituted norms and beliefs. Agency is accomplished within the framework of institutions but these institutions per se are not once and for all given but are instead recursively both shaped by and shaping individual action. Institutional work as a theoretical construct therefore opens up for a more affirmative view of agency without ignoring that such agencies are always firmly grounded in institutional fields. When agents act, they act within institutional fields yet these fields are not determinate structures but are instead flexible and malleable enough to respond and adapt to the agent's behavior and actions.

The field of ART and reproductive medicine is grounded in an intimate expertise of the elementary processes of biological and human reproduction. These processes are what Searle (1995) calls *brute facts*, biomedical processes that operate outside of human influence. In contrast, what Searle calls *institutional facts*, e.g., ideas regarding what are "normal families" and "what is natural" and what is not, that is, ideas that strongly influence the legal and regulatory framework of ART and reproductive medicine, complement the brute facts. Creating possibilities for the largest number of human beings to take advantage of ART and reproductive medicine demand that brute and institutional facts are co-aligned and harmonized, and based on the understanding that there are certain things that can be done and that we want to be done, and certain things that we at least for the time being cannot do regardless of our own beliefs because such practices are not supported by regulatory frameworks and policies. The case of ART and reproductive medicine adds to the stock of institutional theory based studies of this co-alignment work. The case study has specifically demonstrated how biomedicine in the field of assisted reproduction is torn between two end-points on a continuum, where the one end-point is the capacity to do anything practically possible regardless of social beliefs, norms, and the consequences, and the other end-point being a most strict use of the therapies in an attempt to not intervene into the naturally given order of things.

Various actors conduct forms of institutional work from the vantage point of different positions on this continuum. Some actually do think that "baby-markets" should be unregulated to protect individual rights of enterprising and therefore advocate far-reaching deregulatory programs. More moderate agents may advocate the value of a more strict monitoring of the practices to e.g., protect certain groups from being exploited. To the other extreme, there may be e.g., religious groups that reject the reproductive medicine program altogether on the basis of ethical and religious convictions. The study of ART and reproductive medicine thus stresses both the importance of agency in institutional fields while recognizing the centrifugal and centripetal forces that operate in such fields, where some groups embrace all novel possibilities while others see no value in such practices. Ultimately, the study therefore contributes to the understanding of how institutional work is an ongoing and ceaseless activity to create and respond to e.g., new biomedical possibilities and emerging demands being made. Institutional fields are therefore dynamic and changing, in a constant state of flux and renewal and continuously adapting to various stakeholders' expectations and claims.

Contribution to ART studies

Much if not most of the research on ART and reproductive medicine has been conducted in the social sciences and outside of the management studies tradition of research. Sociologists, anthropologists, gender and feminist theorists, science and technology researchers, and political scientists are some of the disciplinary categories of social scientists that have examined the consequences of ART and reproductive medicine. Many of these studies have highlighted important aspects of the new biomedical possibilities and their consequences for human societies. At times, even the economic consequences, e.g., market-making and pricing issues, have been emphasized, but by and large ART and reproductive medicine have been examined from a certain favored theoretical perspective. The present study has aimed to locate ART and reproductive medicine in an institutional field wherein not only social beliefs and practices matter and shape the collective understanding of ART and reproductive medicine but where the day-to-day management and regulatory control of clinical practices is one factor to consider. Social scientists often have a propensity to focus on what is conspicuous, spectacular, and extraordinary, leading to a relatively mild interest for processes of "normalization," i.e., in this case, the work done to institutionalize clinical practices in everyday routines, standard operation procedures, formalized calculative practices, and human resource management work.

Human beings have a natural curiosity that is triggered by novel ideas and changing rules of the game, but much of the accomplishments in everyday social life in late modernity are dependent on the structuring and management of these novel ideas. Processes of e.g., commodification are generally treated as dull or even a source of criticism, but for the wider public the capacity to integrate and commodify a set of previously disjointed clinical practices, medical examinations, tools and technologies, etc., into a standardized therapy package (say, an IVF cycle) is what makes the wondrous accomplishments of brilliant scientists and visionaries ultimately accessible. Bob Edwards was awarded the Nobel Prize in Medicine and Physiology in 2010, perhaps the highest credential offered in biomedicine, but his ground-breaking work was effectively accomplished by the in many cases faceless clinicians, regulators, policy-makers, and managers that structured the generic biomedical know-how into routine work and standard operation procedures.

Star (1999) reminds us that boring things (such as infrastructures, in her case) could be quite exciting if they are examined in their full complexity and within their broader social context. The challenge is just to be able to recognize what escapes our everyday gaze, what we take for granted and what we regard as insignificant. If there is one strength in the management studies perspective, and perhaps even more so in the accounting literature, it is this view that recognizes what other disciplines may regard as boring and unworthy of scholarly attention. While a term like commodification, burdened by its Marxist connotations, is often used in passing as the process wherein something becomes subject to market transactions, management researchers regard this black box of product and service creation as the very act where know-how and expertise are brought to the wider public through market transactions. In other words, while e.g., anthropologists and feminist scholars may shed light on very important issues pertaining to the use of ART and the role of reproductive medicine in contemporary society, they also tend to turn a blind eye to the work to actually produce these clinical practices at a cost level that makes this expertise available for a larger category of social actors.

The study of ART and reproductive medicine is thus not only subject to critical reflection and theoretical analyses, but also needs to be understood as a source of economic venturing and the tinkering taking place in the clinics, in regulatory agencies, in research laboratories, and elsewhere to actively stabilize therapies that can be priced and brought to reproductive market. The organization theory and management studies perspective thus adds to the social science literature on ART and reproductive medicine the practical perspective of how markets and economic activities are the *sine qua non* of health care innovation work and biomedical research. This work may be regarded as dull, uneventful, somewhat "grey," but it is an important process in bringing research work to its end-users, and often demands struggles and much hard work from the actors involved. Management scholars do not fear dull things, and that is one of their merits.

Contribution to policy-making

Social scientists and representatives of the economic sciences should be wary of the risks of making ultracrepidarian recommendations, i.e. of operating outside of one's own domain of expertise. Economists are, for instance, frequently accused of regarding themselves as being in the position to give policy recommendations on the basis of analyses of empirical data and abstract theoretical models including a not negligible amount of assumptions regarding e.g., human preferences and ways of thinking. Anyway, after collecting a set of data it is perhaps not only a privilege but also a duty to articulate some policy implications to help regulators and politicians make their tricky decisions.

The most conspicuous concern during the first decades of functional IVF therapies was the exclusion of lesbian couples and single women. In the former case, it is complicated to identify any other explanatory factor than the sheer discrimination of homosexual women on the basis of heteronormative beliefs and traditions. As the legal status of women as full citizens with the right to vote in public elections, and so forth, is less than 100 years old, and the female sexuality has been a constant source of anxieties and concerns, it is little wonder from a cultural and historical perspective that lesbian women would initially be treated as a problematic deviation from heteronormative standards. What is more complicated to understand is why it took the state of Sweden more than 25 years to make lesbian couples eligible for IVF therapy. Sweden is a country that takes pride in being at the forefront of gender equality and generally embraces new scientific contributions and possibilities, so the apparent discrimination of lesbian couples remains if not a conundrum at least something that historians may be able to explain. However, that issue was resolved in 2006.

The case of single women is perhaps even more complicated as there are no heteronormative beliefs regarding sexual preferences and lifestyles at play in this case. When this book was written in the 2014–2015 period, the legal framework was changed to include single women from July 1, 2015, so this concern has also to some extent been handled after three decades of IVF therapies. Still, the idea of single women not being eligible for medical assistance to become parents primarily violated the norm that all children should have two parents. This norm had limited support in the existing research literature, suggesting that children growing up with one parent are not disadvantaged vis-à-vis children growing up with two parents. The case of illness and death of the one single parent is a factor to consider but in such unfortunate cases, there are often extended families that can step forward to take custody of children.

In addition to the "it takes two parents to make a family" norm, single women were not of necessity infertile at all in the first place. In the case of sub-fertility or infertility of couples seeking medical assistance, there is a record of either an inability to become pregnant or miscarriages. Single women who consider seeking assistance do not of necessity have such concerns. Their concern is the access to sperm to conceive a child. This makes the health care apparatus and the health care policy, already from the beginning concerned with the question of whether infertility is a medical condition or not, even more skeptical towards single women. They are not able to live up to the nuclear family ideal, nor are they suffering from any medical condition, so why should they be catered for? Yet, the policies also made it impossible even to pay the market price of the treatment for single women, since it was illegal to conduct the treatment without evidence of a long-term partner.

One policy implication on the basis of the two cases of lesbian couples and single women is to carefully institute mechanisms that enable a critical and self-reflexive view of the preconceived ideas and norms of e.g., regulators, policy-makers, and politicians that are in charge of policy-making decisions. While the idea that the "best interest of the unborn child" – the guiding principle for e.g., IVF policies in Sweden – is a credible declaration, it also invites conservative and homegrown theories regarding the "best interests" parts of the policy declaration to be more influential than was perhaps intended. Following a liberal tradition of thought, it is not for politicians to be opinionated about whether, for instance, two women are friends or lovers but they should instead ensure that individuals that want to become parents should be given an equal chance without having to testify to e.g., their sexual preferences before a tribunal. In the case of subsidized ART to single women, policy-makers should self-critically assess where the level of generosity of the public health care sector should be and to weigh the social benefits of single women becoming parents in relation to the situation where they fail. An elaborate analysis of the costs and benefits of a more generous policy will possibly reveal that the social and economic benefits overshadow the costs. In addition, the state of Sweden would no longer promote the medical tourism that today benefits Denmark and Finland, both enacting more liberal legislation regarding the rights of single women.

When it comes to the case of the predicament of gay men and the issue of gestational surrogacy, it is not easy to formulate any policy recommendations on the basis of the present study. The question of commercial gestational surrogacy is a most complex question that includes a number of political, ethical, social, and economic issues. The bioethical advisory board has decided to open up the discussion regarding the possibilities for altruistic surrogacy, and for the time being this is perhaps the best way to approach this most difficult issue. It is easy to feel a great deal of sympathy for gay couples being excluded from parenting but commercial gestational surrogacy should perhaps not be justified on such grounds alone since it also involves the needs of other groups in society. Only the future will tell whether a more liberal view of commercial gestational surrogacy will be recognized in the wider public in the future, gradually overcoming the predominant beliefs that most things can be subject to legal agreement, pricing and monetary compensation (e.g., egg donations) but not the female reproductive capabilities. Under all conditions, the selling of eggs and sperm is seen differently than the selling of gestational services but the line of demarcation between the two is far from evident for everyone. Retrieving eggs from the ovaries is also somewhat risky for the female donor, and yet it is permitted by law in Sweden, but pregnancies are not permitted to be sold on the market for primarily medical reasons, making some female ordeals open for market transactions while others are not. But as has already been said, the issue of commercial gestational surrogacy is not a question that should be handled without great care about all perspectives of relevance.

By and large, the Swedish embedded liberalism model with private and public clinics competing in the market and with quite strict regulatory control seem credible and efficient in both securing a good quality of the therapy and to enable competition and renewal. Minor issues regarding e.g., the inability to establish age standards for the different health care regions needs to be further addressed, but the present study adds little new to this ongoing discussion. Swedish ART and reproductive medicine seem to be competitive and to remain vital also at this stage when it is coming of age.

Summary and conclusion

The expression "to make the future" through scientific work is most suitable for reproductive medicine. Indeed, the future is practically made as a new generation of babies is born. The future of ART and reproductive medicine is quite another matter, today operating at the level where roughly 50 percent of the patients seeking assistance are fulfilling the goal of becoming parents. As some of the clinicians argued, few other medical fields and therapeutic areas would take pride in failing in 50 percent of the cases. However, a more forgiving attitude would suggest that despite the remarkable advancement of experimental medicine, it may still be the case that the human biological organism and its reproductive capacities remain concealed in large parts to us, and that future research may give us important knowledge that can help us understand the intricate mechanisms of how human life is created. In practical terms, beyond these grand declarations about revealing the mysteries of life, ART and reproductive medicine is an organized activity located in institutional fields. In many cases the activities are conducted on the basis of commercial interests and considerations, but balanced by monitoring of quality and safety of the patients. This everyday life production of health care services may be less intriguing and may include a lower amount of spectacular events, but still constitute the core of the professional work that structure the institutional field. Being able to shift in focus from what is aimed at creating our biomedical and reproductive futures in scientific communities and what happens in the clinics, the laboratories, among politicians and interest groups is important for understanding how institutional fields are created, maintained, and disrupted by forms of institutional work conducted at various points in time and in various quarters.

Bibliography

Abdelal, R. (2007), *Capital rules: The construction of the global finance*, Cambridge: Harvard University Press.

Abraham, J. (2010), Pharmaceuticalization of society in context: Theoretical, empirical, and health dimensions, *Sociology*, 44(4): 603–622.

Abraham, J. and Davis, C. (2009), Drug evaluation and the permissive principle: Continuities and contradictions between standards and practice in antidepressant regulation, *Social Studies of Science*, 39(4): 569–598.

Abraham, J. and Reed, T. (2002), Progress, innovation and regulatory science in drug development: The politics of international standard-setting, *Social Studies of Science*, 32(3): 337–369.

Aglietta, M. and Rebérioux, A. (2005), *Corporate governance adrift: A critique of shareholder value*, Cheltenham: Edward Elgar.

Akerlof, G.A. and Shiller, R.J. (2009), *Animal spirits: How human psychology drives the economy, and why it matters for global capitalism*, Princeton and London: Princeton University Press.

Almeling, R. (2007), Selling genes, selling gender; Egg agencies, sperm banks, and the medical market in genetic material, *American Sociological Review*, 73(3): 319–340.

Almeling, R. (2011), *Sex cells: The medical market for eggs and sperm*, Berkeley, Los Angeles and London: University of California Press.

Ansari, S. and Phillips, N. (2011), Text me! New consumer practices and change in organizational fields, *Organization Science*, 22(6): 1579–1599.

Argyris, C. and Schön, D.A. (1978), *Organizational learning: A theory of action perspective*, Reading, MA: Addison-Wesley.

Aristotle (1986), *De Anima*, London: Penguin.

Ashcraft, K.L., Kuhn, T.R., and Cooren, F. (2009), Constitutional amendments: "Materializing" organizational communication, *Academy of Management Annals*, 3(1): 1–64.

Ashford, N., Ayers, C., and Stone, R. (1985), Using regulation to change the market for innovation, *Harvard Environment Law Review*, 9(2): 419–466.

Aspers, P. (2010), *Orderly fashion: A sociology of markets*, Princeton: Princeton University Press.

Atkinson, P. and Coffrey, A. (2003), Revisiting the relationship between participant observations and interviewing, in Gubrium, J.F. and Holstein, J.A., eds., (2003), *Postmodern interviewing*, London, Thousand Oaks and New Delhi: Sage, pp. 109–122.

Bailey, A. (2011), Reconceiving surrogacy: Toward a reproductive justice account of Indian surrogacy, *Hypatia*, 26(4): 715–741.

Banerjee, S. and Basu, S. (2009), Rent a womb: Surrogate selection, investment incentives and contracting, *Journal of Economic Behavior & Organization*, 69(3): 260–273.

Baradwaj, A. and Glasner, P. (2009), *Local cells, global science: The rise of embryonic stem cell research in India*, London and New York: Routledge.

Baron, J.N., Dobbin, F.R., and Devereaux Jennings, P. (1986), War and peace: The evolution of modern personnel administration in U.S. industry, *American Journal of Sociology*, 92: 350–383.

Battilana, J. (2006), Agency and institutions: The enabling role of individuals' social position, *Organization*, 13(5): 653–675.

Battilana, J. and D'Aunno, T. (2009), Institutional work and the paradox of embedded agency, in Lawrence, T.B., Suddaby, R. and Leca, B. (2009), *Institutional work: Actors and agency in institutional studies of organization*, Cambridge: Cambridge University Press, pp. 31–58.

Bechky, B.A. (2003), Object lessons: Workplace artifacts as representations of occupational jurisdiction, *American Journal of Sociology*, 109(3): 720–752.

Becker, G. (2000), *The elusive embryo: How women and men approach new reproductive technologies*, Berkeley, Los Angeles and London: University of California Press.

Becker, H.S. (1996), The epistemology of qualitative research, in Jessor, R., Colby, A., and Shweder, R.A. (1996), *Ethnography and human development; Context and meaning in social inquiry*, Chicago and London: The university of Chicago Press, pp. 53–71.

Bedu, N. and Montalban, M. (2014), Analysing the uneven development of private equity in Europe: Legal origins and diversity of capitalism, *Socio-Economic Review*, 12(1): 33–70.

Bennett, J. (2010), *Vibrant matter: A political ecology of things*, Durham and London: Duke University Press.

Bensaude-Vincent, B. (2007), Nanobots and nanotubes: Two alternative biomimetic paradigms of nanotechnology, in Riskin, J. ed., (2007), *Genesis redux: Essays in the history and philosophy of artificial life*, Chicago and London: University of Chicago Press, pp. 211–236.

Bensaude-Vincent, B. and Stengers, I. ([1993] 1996), *A history of chemistry*, trans. by Deborah van Dam, Cambridge and London: Harvard University Press.

Berg, M. and Bowker, G. (1997), The multiple bodies of the medial record: Toward a sociology of an artefact, *Sociological Quarterly*, 38: 511–535.

Berman, E. (2012), *Creating the market university: How academic science became an economic engine*, Princeton and Oxford: Princeton University Press.

Bernard, C. ([1865] 1957), *An introduction to the study of experimental medicine*, trans. by Henry Copley Greene, New York: Dover.

Berube, D.M. (2006), *Nano-hype: The truth behind the nanotechnology buzz*, New York: Prometheus Books.

Birke, L. (2012), Animal bodies in the production of scientific knowledge: Modelling medicine, *Body & Society*, 18(3&4): 156–178.

Bjørkeng, K., Clegg, S., and Pistis, T. (2009), Becoming (a) practice, *Management Learning*, 40(2): 145–159.

Black, D. (2014), An aesthetics of the invisible: Nanotechnology and informatic matter, *Theory, Culture & Society*, 31(1): 99–121.

Blech, J. (2006), *Inventing disease and pushing pills: Pharmaceutical companies and the medicalization of normal life*, trans. By Gisela Wallor Hajjar, London and New York: Routledge.

Blinder, A.S. (2013), *When the music stopped: The financial crisis, the response, and the work ahead*, New York: Penguin.

Block, F. and Keller, M.R. (2009), Where do innovations come from? Transformations in the US economy, 1970–2006, *Socio-Economic Review*, 7(3): 459–483.

Bourdieu, P. (1977), *Outline of a theory of practice*, Cambridge: Cambridge University Press.

Bourdieu, P. (2005), *The economic structures of society*, Cambridge: Polity Press.

Bourdieu, P. and Wacquant, L.J.D. (1992), *An invitation to reflexive sociology*, Chicago and London: The University of Chicago Press.

Bozanic, Z., Dirsmith, M.W., and Huddart, S. (2012), The social constitution of regulation: The endogenization of insider trading laws, *Accounting, Organizations and Society*, 37(7): 461–481.

Braidotti, Rosi, (2006), *Transpositions: On Nomadic Ethics*, Cambridge and Malden: Polity Press.

Braidotti, R. (2008), In spite of the times: The postsecular turn in feminism, *Theory, Culture & Society*, 25(6): 1–24.

Bratton, W.W. and Wachter, M.L. (2010), The case against shareholder empowerment, *Pennsylvania Law Review*, 160(1): 69–168.

Briggs, L. (2010), Reproductive technology: Of labor and markets, *Feminist Studies*, 36(2): 359–374.

Brint, S. (1994), *In the age of experts: The changing role of professionals in politics and public life*, Princeton: Princeton University Press.

Brown, N. and Kraft, A. (2006), Blood ties: Banking the stem cell promise, *Technology Analysis & Strategic Management*, 18(3): 313–327.

Brown, N. and Michael, M. (2003), A sociology of expectations: Retrospecting prospects and prospecting retrospects, *Technology Analysis and Strategic Management*, 15(1): 3–18.

Brown, W. (2006), American nightmare: Neoliberalism, neoconservatism, and de-democratization, *Political Theory*, 34(6): 690–714.

Bud, R. (1983), *The uses of life: A history of biotechnology*, Cambridge: Cambridge University Press.

Bullough, V.L. (1994), *Science in the bedroom: A history of sex research*, New York: Basic Books.

Burgin, A. (2012), *The great persuasion: Reinventing free markets since the Depression*, Cambridge: Harvard University Press.

Bynum, W.E. (1994), *Science and the practice of medicine in the Nineteenth century*, Cambridge: Cambridge University Press.

Cahn, N. (2010), Reproducing dreams, in Goodwin, Michele Bratcher, ed., (2010), *Baby markets: Money and the new politics of creating families*, Cambridge: Cambridge University Press, pp. 147–163.

Callon, M. (1981), Some Elements of a Sociology of Translation: Domestication of the Scallops and the Fishermen of St Brieuc Bay, in Knorr-Cetina, K. and Cicourel, A.V., eds., (1981), *Advances in social theory and methodology: Toward an integration of micro and macro sociologies*, London: Routledge and Kegan Paul.

Cambrosio, A., Keating, P., Schlich, T., and Weisz, G. (2006), Regulatory objectivity and the generation and management of evidence in medicine, *Social Science & Medicine*, 63(1): 189–199.

Campbell, N. and Saren, M. (2010), The primitive, technology and horror: A posthuman biology, *Ephemera*, 10(2): 152–176.

Canguilhem, G. (2008), *Knowledge of life*, trans. by Stefano Geroulanos, and Daniela Ginsburg, New York: Fordham University Press.

Caroll, B., Levy, L. and Richmond, D. (2008), Leadership as practice: Challenging the competency paradigm, *Leadership*, 4(4): 363–379.

Carr-Saunders, A.M. and Wilson, P.A. (1933), *The professions*, Oxford: Clarendon Press. (Parts II–V)

Carruthers, B.G. and Stinchcombe, A.L. (1999), The social structure of liquidity flexibility, markets and states, *Theory and Society*, 28: 353–382.

Carter, C., Clegg, S.R., and Kornberger, M. (2008), Strategy as practice?, *Strategic Organization*, 6(1): 83–99.

Champy, F. (2006), Professional discourses under the pressures of economic values: The case of French architects, *Current Sociology*, 54(4): 649–661.

Changeux, J.-P. (2004), *The physiology of truth: Neuroscience and human knowledge*, Boston: Belknap Press of Harvard University Press.

Cheal, D. (1988), *The gift economy*, London and New York: Routledge.

Cherry, M.J. (2005), *Kidney for sale by owner: Transplantation and the market*, Washington: Georgetown University Press.

Chesbrough, H.W. (2003), *Open innovation: The new imperative for creating and profiting from technology*, Boston: Harvard Business School Press.

Choi, H. and Mody, C.C.M. (2009), The long history of molecular electronics: Microelectronics origins of nanotechnology, *Social Studies of Science*, 39(1): 11–50.

Clarke, A. (1990), Controversy and the development of reproductive sciences, *Social Problems*, 37(1): 18–27.

Clarke, A.E. (1998), *Disciplining reproduction: Modernity, American life sciences, and the problem of sex*, Berkeley: University of California Press.

Clarke, A.E., Mamo, L., Fishman, J.R., Shim, J.K., and Fosket, J.R. (2003), Biomedicalization: Technoscientific transformations of health, illness, and U.S. biomedicine, *American Sociological Review*, 68: 161–194.

Clarke, A.E., Shim, J.K., Mamo, L., Fosket, J.R., and Fishman J.R. (2010a), Biomedicalization: technoscientific transformations of health, illness, and U.S. biomedicine, in Clarke, A.E., Mamo, L., Fosket, J.R., Fishman, J.R., and Shim, J.K., eds., (2010), *Biomedicalization: Technoscience, Health, Illness in the U.S.*, Durham and London: Duke University Press, pp. 47–87.

Coates, J.C. IV (2007), The goals and promise of the Sarbanes–Oxley Act, *Journal of Economic Perspectives*, 21(1): 91–116.

Cockburn, I.M. and Stern, S. (2010), Finding the endless frontier: Lessons from the life sciences innovation system for technology policy, *Capitalism and Society*, 5(1): 1–48.

Cohan, W.D. (2011), *Money and power: How Goldman Sachs came to rule the world*, London: Allen Lane and New York: Anchor Books.

Cohen, M.D., March, J.G., and Olsen, J.P. (1972), A garbage can model of organizational choice, *Administrative Science Quarterly*, 17: 1–25.

Collins, R. (1979), *The credential society*, New York: Academic Press.

Comte, A. (1975), *Auguste Comte and positivism: Essential writings*, Ed. by Gertrud Lenzer, New York: Harper Torchbooks.

Conrad, P. (2007), *The medicalization of society*, Baltimore: Johns Hopkins University Press.

Cooper, M. (2008), *Life as surplus: Biotechnology and capitalism in the neoliberal era*, Seattle and London: The University of Washington Press.

Cooren, F. (2004), Textual agency: How texts do things in organizational settings, *Organization*, 11(3): 373–393.

Corra, M. and Willer, D. (2002), The gatekeeper, *Sociological Theory*, 20(2): 180–207.

Crossan, M.M. and Apaydin, M. (2010), A multi-dimensional framework of organizational innovation: A systematic review of the literature, *Journal of Management Studies*, 47(6): 1154–1191.

Crotty, J. (2008), If financial market competition is intense, why are financial firm profits so high? Reflections on the current "golden age" of finance, *Competition & Change*, 12(2): 167–183.

Crouch, C. (2011), *The strange non-death of neo-liberalism*, Cambridge: Polity.

Currie, G., Lockett, A., Finn, R., Martin, G., and Waring, J. (2012), Institutional work to maintain professional power: Recreating the model of medical professionalism, *Organization Studies*, 33(7): 937–962.

Cussins, C. (1996), Ontological choreography: Agency through objectification in infertility clinics, *Social Studies of Science*, 26: 575–610.

Cussins, C. (1998), Reproducing reproduction: Techniques of normalization and naturalization in infertility clinics, in Franklin, S. and Ragoné, H., eds., (1998), *Reproducing reproduction: Kinship, power, and technological innovation*, Philadelphia: University of Pennsylvania Press, pp. 86–101.

Daft, R.L. and Weick, K.E. (1984), Toward a model of organizations as interpretation systems, *Academy of Management Review*, 9(2): 284–295.

Das, V. (2000), The practice of organ transplants: Networks, documents, translations, in Lock, M., Youg, A., and Cambrosio, A., eds., (2000), *Living and working with new medical technologies: Intersections of inquiry*, Cambridge: Cambridge University Press, pp. 263–287.

Daston, L. (1995), The moral economy of science, *Osiris*, 10: 2–24.

Davey, S.M., Brennan, M., Meenan, B.J., and McAdam, R. (2011), Innovation in the medical device sector: An open business model approach for high-tech small firms, *Technology Analysis & Strategic Management*, 23(8): 807–824.

David, Matthew, ed., (2006), *Case study research, Vol. 1*, London, Thousand Oaks and New Delhi: Sage.

Davies, G. (2013), Mobilizing experimental life: Spaces of becoming with mutant mice, *Theory Culture Society*, 30(7/8): 129–153.

Davis, G.F., Diekmann, K.A., and Tinsley, C. (1994), The decline and fall of the conglomerate firm in the 1980s: The deinstitutionalization of an organization form, *American Sociological Review*, 59: 547–570.

De Roover, R. (1974c), The scholastic attitude toward trade and entrepreneurship, in De Roover, Raymond, (1974), *Banking business, and economic thought in early modern Europe: Selected studies of Raymond de Roover*, Kirshner, J., ed., Chicago and London: The University of Chicago Press, pp. 336–345.

Dickenson, D. (2008), *Body shopping: The economy fuelled by flesh and blood*, Oxford: Oneworld.

Dilthey, W. (1988), *Introduction to the human sciences: An attempt to lay a foundation for the study of society and history*, Detroit: Wayne State University Press.

DiMaggio, P. (1987), Classification in Art, *American Sociological Review*, 52(4): 440–455.

DiMaggio, P. and Louch, H. (1998), Socially embedded consumer transactions: For what kinds of purchases do people most often use networks, *American Sociological Review*, 63(5): 619–637.

DiMaggio, P. and Powell, W.W. (1983), The iron cage revisited: Institutional isomorphism and collective rationality in organizational fields, *American Sociological Review*, 48(2): 147–160.

Dobbin, F. and Dowd, T.J. (2000), The market that antitrust built: Public policy, private coercion, and railroad acquisitions, 1825 to 1922, *American Sociological Review*, 65(5): 631–657.

Dobbin, F. and Sutton, J.R. (1998), The strength of a weak state: The rights revolution and the rise of human resources management divisions, *American Journal of Sociology*, 104(2): 441–476.

Douglas, M. (1986), *How institutions think*, London: Routledge and Kegan Paul.

Driessens, O. (2013), Celebrity capital: Redefining celebrity using field theory, *Theory and Society*, 42(5): 543–560.

Du Gay, P., Millo, Y., and Tuck, P. (2012), Making government liquid: Shifts in governance using financialisation as a political device, *Environment and Planning C: Government and Policy*, 30(6): 1083–1099.

Dumit, J. (2012), *Drugs for life: How pharmaceutical companies define our health*, Durham and London: Duke University Press.

Dunn, M.R. and Jones, C. (2010), Institutional logics and institutional pluralism: The contestation of care and science logics in medical education, 1967–2005, *Administrative Science Quarterly*, 55: 114–149.

Durkheim, E. (1895/1938), *The Rules of Sociological Method*, Glencoe: Free Press.

Durkheim, É. and Mauss, M. (1963), *Primitive classification*, trans. by Rodney Needham, Chicago: The University of Chicago Press.

Edelman, L.B. (1990), Legal environments and organizational governance: The expansion of due process in the American workplace, *American Journal of Sociology*, 95(6): 1401–1440.

Edelman, L. (1992), Legal ambiguity and symbolic structures: Organizational meditation of civil rights law, *American Journal of Sociology*, 97: 1531–1576.

Edelman, L.B. and Suchman, M.C. (1997), The legal environment of organizations, *Annual Review of Sociology*, 23: 479–515.

Edelman, L.B., Fuller, S.R., and Mara-Drita, I. (2001), Diversity rhetoric and the managerialization of law, *American Journal of Sociology*, 106(6): 1589–1641.

Edwards, R.G. (2001), The bumpy road to human in-vitro fertilization, *Nature Medicine*, 13(7): 1091–1094.

Elias, N. (1978), *The civilizing process*, Oxford: Blackwell.

Elster, N.R. (2010), Egg donation for research and reproduction: The compensation conundrum, in Goodwin, Michele Bratcher, ed., (2010), *Baby markets: Money and the new politics of creating families*, Cambridge: Cambridge University Press, pp. 226–236.

Emirbayer, M. and Mische, A. (1998), What is agency?, *American Journal of Sociology*, 103(4): 962–1023.

Ertman, M. (2010), The upside of baby markets, in Goodwin, Michele Bratcher, ed., (2010), *Baby markets: Money and the new politics of creating families*, Cambridge: Cambridge University Press, pp. 23–40.

Eyal, G. (2013), For a sociology of expertise: The social origins of the autism epidemic, *American Journal of Sociology*, 118(4): 863–907.

Fannin, M. (2013), The hoarding economy of endometrial stem cell storage, *Body & Society*, 19(4): 32–60.

Faulkner, A. (2012), Law's performativities: Shaping the emergence of regenerative medicine through European Union legislation, *Social Studies of Science*, 42(5): 753–774.

Feldman, M.S. and Pentland, B.T. (2003), Reconceptualizing organization routines as a source of flexibility and change, *Administrative Science Quarterly*, 48: 94–118.

Feldman, M.S. and Pentland, B.T. (2005), Organizational routines and the macro-actors, in Czarniawska, B. and Hernes, T. (2005), *Actor-network theory and organizing*, Malmö: Liber and Copenhagen: Copenhagen Business School Press, pp. 91–111.

Ferguson, P. (2004), *Accounting for taste: The triumph of French cuisine*, Chicago and London: The University of Chicago Press.

Ferguson, P. (2006), *Accounting for taste: The triumph of French cuisine*, Chicago: University of Chicago Press.

Fine, G.A. (2007), *Authors of the storm: Meteorologists and the culture of prediction*, Chicago and London: The University of Chicago Press.

Fligstein, N. (1987), The interorganizational power struggle: Rise of financial personnel to top leadership in large corporations, *American Sociological Review*, 52(1): 44–58.

Fligstein, N. (1990), *The transformation of corporate control*, Cambridge and London: Harvard University Press.

Fligstein, N. (1996), Markets as politics: A political-cultural approach to market institutions, *American Sociological Review*, 61(4): 656–673.

Fligstein, N. (2001), *The architecture of markets*, Princeton: Princeton University Press.

Fligstein, N. and Choo, J. (2005), Law and corporate governance, *Annual Review of Law and Social Science*, 1: 61–84.

Fligstein, N. and McAdam, D. (2012), *A theory of fields*, New York and Oxford: Oxford University Press.

Foucault, M. (1973), *The birth of the clinic*, London: Routledge.

Foucault, M., (1978), *The history of sexuality, Vol. 1: The will to knowledge*, New York: Vintage.

Foucault, M. (1988), *The history of sexuality, Vol. 2: The use of pleasure*, London: Penguin.

Foucault, M. (1990), *The history of sexuality, Vol. 3: The care of the self*, London: Penguin.

Fourcade, M. (2011), Cents and sensibility: Economic valuation and the nature of "nature," *American Journal of Sociology*, 116(6): 1721–1777.

Franklin, S. (1998), Making miracles: Scientific progress and the facts of life, in Franklin, S. and Ragoné, H., eds., (1998), *Reproducing reproduction: Kinship, power, and technological innovation*, Philadelphia: University of Pennsylvania Press, pp. 102–117.

Franklin, S. (2005), Stem Cell R Us: Emergent life forms and the global biological, in Ong, A. and Collier, S.J., eds., (2008), *Global assemblages: Technology, politics, and ethics as anthropological problems*, Malden and Oxford: Blackwell, pp. 59–78.

Franklin, S. (2014), *Biological relatives: IVF, stem cells, and the future of kinship*, Durham and London: Duke University Press.

Franklin, S. and Roberts, C. (2006), *Born and made: An ethnography of preimplantation genetic diagnosis*, Princeton and London: Princeton University Press.

Friedlander, R. and Alford, R.R. (1991), Bringing society back in: Symbols, practices and institutional contradictions, in DiMaggio, P.J., and Powell, W.W. (1991), *The new institutionalism in organizational snalysis*, Chicago: University of Chicago Press, pp. 232–263.

Friedman, J. and Kraus, W. (2012), *Engineering the financial crisis: Systemic risk and the failure of regulation*, Philadelphia: University of Pennsylvania Press.

Friedman, M. ([1962] 2002), *Capitalism and freedom*, 4th edn, Chicago and London: The University of Chicago Press.

Friese, C. and Clarke, A.E. (2012), Transposing bodies of knowledge and technique: Animal models at work in reproductive sciences, *Social Studies of Science*, 42(1): 31–52.

Fujimura, J.H. (1996), *Crafting science: A sociohistory of the quest for the genetics of cancer*, Cambridge, Mass.: Harvard University Press.

Fujimura, J.H. (2005), Postgenomic futures: Translating across the machine-nature border in systems biology, *New Genetics and Society*, 24(2): 195–225.

Fujimura, J.H. (2006), Sex genes: A critical sociomaterial approach to the politics and molecular genetics of sex determination, *Signs*, 32(1): 49–82.

Gay, P. (2001), *Schnitzler's century: The making of middle-class culture, 1815–1914*, London: Allen Lane.

Gershon, I. (2011), Neoliberal agency, *Current Anthropology*, 52(4): 537–555.

Gibbert, M., Ruigrok, W., and Wicki, B. (2008), What passes as a rigorous case study?, *Strategic Management Journal*, 29: 1465–1474.

Giddens, A. (1984), *The constitution of society*, Chicago: The University of Chicago Press.

Ginsburg, F. and Rapp, R. (1991), The politics of reproduction, *Annual Review of Anthropology*, 20: 311–343.

Glasner, P. (2005), Banking on immortality: Exploring the stem cell supply chain from embryo to therapeutic applications, *Current Sociology*, 45(2): 355–366.

Goodwin, M.B. (2010), Baby markets, in Goodwin, M.B., ed., (2010), *Baby markets: Money and the new politics of creating families*, Cambridge: Cambridge University Press, pp. 2–22.

Goodwin, M. (2011), Relational markets and justice paradoxes, *Social Research*, 78(3): 829–848.

Goody, J. (1986), *The logic of writing and the organization of society*, Cambridge: Cambridge University Press.

Goslinga-Roy, G. (2000), Body boundaries, fiction of the female self: An ethnography of power, feminism and the reproductive technologies, *Feminist Studies*, 26(1): 113–140.

Gourevitch, P.A. and Shinn, J. (2005), *Political power and corporate control: The new global politics of corporate governance*, Princeton University Press.

Granovetter, M. (1985), Economic action and social structure, *American Journal of Sociology*, 91(3): 481–510.

Greenwood, R., Suddaby, R., and Hinings, C.R. (2002), Theorizing change: The role of professional associations in the transformation of institutional fields, *Academy of Management Journal*, 45(1): 58–80.

Griesemer, J. (2006), Genetics from an evolutionary perspective, in Neumann-Held, E.M. and Rehmann-Sutter, C., eds., (2006), *Genes in development; Re-reading the molecular paradigm*, Durham and London: Duke University Press, pp. 199–237.

Guillén, M.F., Collins, R., England, P., and Meyer, M. (2002), The revival of economic sociology, in Guillén, M.F., Collins, R., England, P., and Meyer, M., eds., (2002), *The new economic sociology: Development in emerging fields*, New York: Russell Sage Foundation, pp. 1–32.

Habermas, J. (2003), *The future of human nature*, Cambridge: Polity Press.

Hacking, I. (2002), *Historical ontology*, Cambridge: Harvard University Press.

Haigh, E. (1984), *Xavier Bichat and the medical theory of the eighteenth century*, London: The Wellcome Institute for the History of Medicine.

Halliday, T.C. and Carruthers, B.G. (2007), The recursivity of law: Global norm making and national lawmaking in the globalization of corporate insolvency regimes, *American Journal of Sociology*, 112(4): 1135–1202.

Hammons, S.A. (2008), Assisted reproductive technologies: Changing conceptions of motherhood?, *Affilia: Journal of Women and Social Work*, 23(3): 270–280.

Harcourt, B.E. (2011), *The illusion of free markets*, Cambridge and London: Harvard University Press.

Harvey, D. (2005), *A brief history of neoliberalism*, New York: Oxford University Press.

Hayek, F., von, (1949), "Free" enterprise and competitive order, in *Individualism and economic order*, London: Routledge and Kegan Paul, pp. 107–118.

Healy, K. (2004), Altruism as an organizational problem: The case of organ procurement, *American Sociological Review*, 69: 387–404.

Hedgecoe, A. (2010), Bioethics and the reinforcement of socio-technical expectations, *Organization*, 17(2): 163–186.

Heilbron, J., Verheul, J., and Quak, S. (2013), The origins and early diffusion of "shareholder value" in the United States, *Theory and Society*, 43(1): 1–22.

Hiatt, S.R. and Park, S. (2013), Lords of the harvest: Third-party influence and regulatory approval of genetically modified organisms, *Academy of Management Journal*, 56(4): 923–944.

High, B. (2009), The recent historiography of American neoconservatism, *The Historical Journal*, 52(2): 475–491.

Hochschild, A.R. (1997), *The time bind: When work becomes home and home becomes work*, New York: Metropolitan Books.

Hochschild, A.R. (2012), *The outsourced self: Intimate life in market times*, New York: Metropolitan Books.

Hoeyer, K. (2009), Tradable body parts? How bone and recycled prosthetic devices acquire a price without forming a "market," *Biosocieties*, 4(2–3): 239–256.

Hoeyer, K., Nexoe, S., Hartlev, M., and Koch, L. (2009), Embryonic entitlements: Stem cell patenting and the co-production of commodities and personhood, *Body & Society*, 15(1): 1–24.

Hogle, L.F. (2009), Pragmatic objectivity and the standardization of engineered tissues, *Social Studies of Science*, 39: 717–742.

Holstein, J.A. and Gubrium, J.F., eds., (2003), *Inside interviewing: New lenses, new concerns*, London, Thousand Oaks and New Delhi: Sage.

Hopkins, M.M., Martin, P.A., Nightingale, P., Kraft, A., and Mahdi, S. (2007), The myth of a biotech revolution: An assessment of technological, clinical and organizational change, *Research Policy*, 36(4): 566–589.

Ikemoto, L.C. (2009), Eggs as capital: Human egg procurement in the fertility industry and the stem cell research enterprise, *Signs*, 34(4): 763–781.

Ikemoto, L.C. (2010), Eggs, nests, and stem cells, in Goodwin, M.B., ed., (2010), *Baby markets: Money and the new politics of creating families*, Cambridge: Cambridge University Press, pp. 237–250.

Ingold, T. (2010), The textility of making, *Cambridge Journal of Economics*, 34: 91–201.

Inhorn, M.C. and Birenbaum-Carmeli, D. (2008), Assisted reproductive technologies and culture change, *Annual Review of Anthropology*, 37: 177–196.

Innes, H.A. ([1950] 1972), *Empire and communications*, 2nd edn., Toronto: University of Toronto Press.

James, W. (1975), *Pragmatism and the meaning of truth*, Cambridge: Harvard University Press.

Jasanoff, S. (2005), The idiom of co-production, in Jasanoff, S., ed., (2005), *States of knowledge: The co-production of science and social order*, London and New York: Routledge, pp. 1–12.

Johnson, M.H. (2011), Robert Edwards: The path to IVF, *Reproductive Biomedicine Online*, 23: 245–262.

Johnson, P. (2010), *Making the market: Victorian origins of corporate capitalism*, Cambridge: Cambridge University Press.

Johnson, T.J. (1972), *Professions and power*, London: Macmillan.

Jones, D.S. (2012), *Masters of the universe: Hayek, Friedman, and the birth of neoliberal politics*, Princeton and Oxford: Princeton University Press.

Jones, R.A.I. (2004), *Soft machines: Nanotechnology and life*, Oxford and New York: Oxford University Press.

Jordan, K. and Lynch, M. (1992), The sociology of a genetic engineering technique: Ritual and rationality in the performance of the "plasmic prep," in Clarke, A.E. and Fujimura, J.H., eds., (1992), *The right tools for the job: At work in twentieth-century life sciences*, Princeton: Princeton University Press, pp. 77–114.

Kant, I. (1952), *The critique of judgement*, trans. by James Creed Meredith, Oxford: Clarendon Press.

Katz, D. and Kahn, R.L. (1966), *The social psychology of organizations*, New York: Wiley.

Kay, L.E. (2000), *Who wrote the book of life? A history of the genetic code*, Stanford and London: Stanford University Press.

Keller, E.F. (2000), *The century of the gene*, Cambridge and London: Harvard University Press.

Keller, E.F. (2002), *Making sense of life: Explaining biological development with models, metaphors, and machines*, Cambridge and London: Harvard University Press.

Keller, E.F. (2010), *The mirage of a space between nature and nurture*, Durham and London: Duke University Press.

Kelly, E. and Dobbin, F. (1999), Civil rights law at work: Sex discrimination and the rise of maternity leave policies, *American Journal of Sociology*, 105(2): 455–492.

Kevles, D.J. (2002), Of mice and money: The story of the world's first animal patent, *Daedalus*, 131(2): 78–88.

Kitchener, M. (2002), Mobilizing the logic of managerialism in professional fields: The case of academic health centre mergers, *Organization Studies*, 23(3): 391–420.

Knorr, C. and Karin, D. (1983), The ethnographic study of scientific work: Towards a constructivist interpretation of science, in Knorr, C., Karin, D., and Mulkay, M., eds., (1983), *Science observed: Perspectives on the social study of science*, London, Beverly Hills and New Delhi: Sage, pp. 115–140.

Kohler, R. (1994), *Lords of the fly: Drosophila genetics and experience of life*, Chicago and London: The University of Chicago Press.

Kohli-Laven, N., Bourret, P., Keating, P., and Cambrosio, A. (2011), Cancer clinical trials in the era of genomic signatures: Biomedical innovation, clinical utility, and regulatory scientific hybrids, *Social Studies of Science*, 41(4): 487–513.

Koyré, A. (1968), *Metaphysics and measurement*, Reading: Gordon and Breach Science Publishers.

Krawiec, K.D. (2010), Price and pretence in baby markets, in Goodwin, M.B., ed., (2010), *Baby markets: Money and the new politics of creating families*, Cambridge: Cambridge University Press, pp. 41–55.

Kvale, S. (1996), *InterViewing*, London, Thousand Oaks and New Delhi: Sage.

Lakoff, A. (2007), The right patients for the drug: Managing the placebo effect in antidepressant trials, *Biosocieties*, 2(1): 57–71.

Lakoff, A. (2012), Diagnostic liquidity: Mental illness and the global trade in DNA, in Sunder Rajan, Kaushik, ed., (2012), *Lively capital*, Durham and London: Duke University Press, pp. 251–278.

Lakoff, A. and Klinenberg, E. (2010), Of risk and pork: Urban security and the politics of objectivity, *Theory and Society*, 39: 502–525.

Landes, E.M. and Posner, RA. (1978), The economics of the baby shortage, *Journal of Legal Studies*, 7: 323–348.

Larson, M.S. (1977), *The rise of professionalism: A sociological analysis*, Berkeley, Los Angeles, and London: University of California Press.

Latimer, J., Featherstone, K., Atkinson, P., Clarke, A., Pilz, D.T., and Shaw, A. (2006), Rebirthing the clinic: The interaction of clinical judgment and genetic technology in the production of medical science, *Science Technology Human Values*, 31(5): 599–630.

Latour, B. (1988), *The pasteurization of France*, trans. by Alan Sheridan and John Law, Cambridge and London: Harvard University Press.

Latour, B. (1995), Joliot: History and physics mixed together, in Serres, M., ed., (1995), *A History of Scientific Thought*, Oxford: Blackwell.

Law, J. (1994), *Organizing modernity*, Oxford and Cambridge: Blackwell.

Lawrence, P.R. and Lorsch, J.W. (1967), *Organization and environment: Managing differentiation and integration*, Boston: Harvard Business School Press.

Lawrence, T., Suddaby, R., and Leca, B. (2009), Introduction: Theorizing and studying institutional work, in Lawrence, T., Suddaby, R., and Leca, B. (2009), *Institutional work: Actors and agency in institutional studies of organization*, Cambridge: Cambridge University Press, pp. 1–27.

Lawrence, T., Suddaby, R., and Leca, B. (2011), Institutions and work: Refocusing institutional studies of organization, *Journal of Management Inquiry*, 20(1): 52–58.

Lawrence, T.B. (2004), Rituals and resistance: Membership dynamics in professional fields, *Human Relations*, 57(2): 113–143.

Lawrence, T.B., Leca, B. and Zilber, T.B. (2013), Institutional work: Current research, new directions and overlooked issues, *Organization Studies*, 34(8): 1023–1033.

Leblebici, H., Salancik, G.R., Copay, A., and King, T. (1991), Institutional change and the transformation of interorganizational fields: An organizational history of the U.S. radio broadcasting system, *Administrative Science Quarterly*, 36: 333–363.

Lemke, T. (2011), *Biopolitics: An advanced introduction*, New York: New York University Press.

Lenoir, T. (1980), Kant, Blumenbach, and vital materialism in German biology, *Isis*, 71(1): 77–108.

Lenoir, T. (1997), *Instituting science: The cultural production of scientific disciplines*, Stanford: Stanford University Press.

Lenoir, T. (1998), Revolution from above: The role of the state in creating the German research system, 1810–1910, *The American Economic Review*, 88(2): 22–27.

Leong, N. (2013), Racial capitalism, *Harvard Law Review*, 126(8): 2152–2226.

Lévi-Strauss, C. (1985), *The view from afar*, trans. by Joachim Neugroshel and Phoebe Hoss, Oxford: Blackwell.

Lewis, J., Atkinson, P., Harrington, J., and Featherstone, K. (2013), Representation and practical accomplishment in the laboratory: When is an animal model *Good-enough*?, *Sociology*, 47(4): 776–792.

Lindblom, C.E. (1959), The science of muddling through, *Public Administration Review*, 19(2): 79–88.

Lock, M. (2002), *Twice dead: Organ transplants and the reinvention of death*, Berkeley. Los Angeles, and London: University of California Press.

Lock, M. (2007), The future is now: Locating biomarkers for dementia, in Burri, R.V. and Dumit, J., eds., (2007), *Biomedicine as culture: Instrumental practices, technoscientific knowledge, and new modes of life*, New York and London: Routledge, pp. 61–85.

Lok, J. (2010), Institutional logics as identity projects, *Academy of Management Journal*, 53(6): 1305–1335.

Longino, H.E. (1992), Knowledge, bodies, and values: Reproductive technologies and their strategic context, *Inquiry*, 35(3/4): 323–340.

Lorenz, C. (2012), If you're so smart, why are you under surveillance? Universities, neoliberalism, and new public management, *Critical Inquiry*, 38: 599–629.

Lounsbury, M., (2008), Institutional rationality and practice variation: New directions in the institutional analysis of practice, *Accounting, Organization and Society*, 33: 349–361.

Löwith, K. (1993), *Max Weber and Karl Marx*, trans. by Hans Hantel, London and New York: Routledge.

Luhmann, N. (1986), *Love as passion: The codification of intimacy*, trans. by Jeremy Gaines and Doris L. Jones, Cambridge: Polity.

Lyotard, J.-F. ([1979] 1984), *The Postmodern Condition: A report on Knowledge*, Manchester: Manchester University Press.

Maguire, S. and Hardy, C. (2009), Discourse and deinstitutionalization: The decline of DDT, *Academy of Management Journal*, 52(1): 148–178.

Mamo, L. (2007), *Queering reproduction: Achieving pregnancy in the age of technoscience*, Durham and London: Duke University Press.

Mandis, S.G. (2013), *What happened to Goldman Sachs: An insider's story of organizational drift and its unintended consequences*, Boston and London: Harvard Business Review Press.

March, J.G. and Olsen, J. (1976), *Ambiguity and choice in organizations*, Oslo: Universitetsforlaget.

Markens, S. (2007), *Surrogate motherhood and the politics of reproduction*, Berkeley and Los Angeles: University of California Press.

Martin, L.J. (2009), Reproductive tourism in the age of globalization, *Globalizations*, 6(2): 249–263.

Martin, L.J. (2010), Anticipating infertility egg freezing, genetic preservation, and risk, *Gender & Society*, 24(4): 526–545.

Martin, L.J. (2014), The world's not ready for this globalizing selective technologies, *Science, Technology & Human Values*, 39(3): 432–455.

Martin, P., Brown, N., and Kraft, A. (2008), From bedside to bench? Communities of promise, translational research and the making of blood stem cell, *Science as Culture*, 23(3): 349–380.

McGoey, L. (2010), Profitable failure: Antidepressant drugs and the triumph of flawed experiments, *History of the Human Sciences*, 23(1): 58–78.

Merton, R.K. (1936), The unanticipated consequences of purposive social action, *American Sociological Review*, 1(6): 894–904.

Meyer, J.W. and Jepperson, R.L. (2000), The "actors" of modern society: The cultural construction of social agency, *Sociological Theory*, 18(1): 100–120.

Meyer, J.W. and Rowan, B. (1977), Institutionalizing organizations: Formal structure as myth and ceremony, *American Journal of Sociology*, 83(2): 340–363.

Meyer, J.W., and Rowan, B. (1977), Institutionalizing organizations: Formal structure as myth and ceremony, *American Journal of Sociology*, 83(2): 340–363.

Meyer, R.E. and Hammerschmid, G. (2006), Changing institutional logics and executive identities: A managerial challenge to public administration in Austria, *American Behavioral Scientist*, 49(7): 1000–1014.

Milburn, C. (2004), Nanotechnology in the age of posthuman engineering: Science fiction as science, in Hayles, N. Katherine, ed., (2005), *Nanoculture: Implications of the new technoscience*, Bristol: Intellect Books, pp. 109–129.

Miller, P. and Rose, N. (1990), Governing economic life, *Economy and Society*, 19(1): 1–31.

Milonakis, D. and Fine, B. (2009), *From political economy to economics: Method, the social and the historical in the evolution of economic theory*, London and New York: Routledge.

Mirowski, P. (2011), *Science-Mart: Privatizing American science*, Cambridge and London: Harvard University Press.

Mirowski, P. (2013), *Never let a serious crisis go to waste: How neoliberalism survived the financial meltdown*, London and New York: Verso.

Mizruchi, M.S. (2010), The American corporate elites and the historical roots of the financial crisis of 2008, *Research in the Sociology of Organizations*, Volume 30B: 103–139.

Mohapatra, S. (2012), Stateless babies & adoption scams: A bioethical analysis of international commercial surrogacy, *Berkeley Journal of International Law*, 30(2): 412–450.

Mol, A. (2002), *The body multiple: Ontology in medical practice*, Durham: Duke University Press.

Monson, I. (2008), Hearing, seeing, and perceptual agency, *Critical Inquiry*, 34, suppl. (Winter 2008): 836–858.

Mowery, D.C. (2009), *Plus ça change*: Industrial R&D in the "third industrial revolution," *Industrial and Corporate Change*, 18(1): 93–108.

Murphy, M. (2013), *Seizing the means of reproduction: Entanglements of feminism, health, and technoscience*, Durham and London: Duke University Press.

Murray, F. (2010), The oncomouse that roared: Hybrid exchanges as a source of distinction at the boundary of overlapping institutions, *American Journal of Sociology*, 116(2): 341–388.

Myers, N. (2008), Molecular embodiments and the body-work of modeling in protein crystallography, *Social Studies of Science*, 38: 163–199.

Neumann-Held, E.M. (2006), Genes-Causes-Codes: Deciphering DNA's ontological privilege, in Neumann-Held, E.M. and Rehmann-Sutter, C., eds., (2006), *Genes in development: Re-reading the molecular paradigm*, Durham and London: Duke University Press, pp. 238–271.

Neumann-Held, E.M. and Rehmann-Sutter, C., eds., (2006), *Genes in development: Re-reading the molecular paradigm*, Durham and London: Duke University Press.

Nicolini, D. (2013), *Practice theory, work, and organization: An introduction*, Oxford and New York: Oxford University Press.

Nicolini, D., Mengis, J., and Swan, J. (2012), Understanding the role of objects in cross-disciplinary collaboration, *Organization Science*, 23(3): 612–629.

Nielsen, M. (2012), *Reinventing discovery: The new era of networked science*, Princeton and Oxford: Princeton University Press.

Nigam, A. and Ocasio, W. (2010), Even attention, environmental sensemaking, and change in institutional logics: An inductive analysis of the effects of public attention to Clinton's health care reform initiative, *Organization Science*, 21(4): 823–841.

Nye, D.E. (1990), *Electrifying America: social meanings of a new technology, 1880–1940*, Cambridge: The MIT Press.

Oberman, M., Wolf, L., and Zettler, P. (2010), Where stem cell research meets abortion politics: Limits on buying and selling human oocytes, in Goodwin, Michele Bratcher, ed., (2010), *Baby markets: Money and the new politics of creating families*, Cambridge: Cambridge University Press, pp. 251–264.

Obstfeld, D. (2005), Social networks, the tertius iungens orientation, and involvement in innovation, *Administrative Science Quarterly*, 50(1): 100–130.

Olson, M. (1965), *The logic of collective action*, Cambridge: Harvard University Press.

Ong, W.J. (1982), *Orality and literacy: The technologizing of the word*, London: Routledge.

Orlikowski, W.J. (2007), Sociomaterial practices: Exploring technology at work, *Organization Studies*, 28(9): 1435–1448.

Owen-Smith, J. (2006), Commercial imbroglios: Proprietary science the contemporary university, in Frickell, S. and Moore, K. eds., (2006), *The new political sociology of science: Institutions, networks and power*, Madison: The University of Wisconsin Press, pp. 63–90.

Owen-Smith, J. and Powell, W.W. (2004), Knowledge networks as channels and conduits: The effects of spillovers in the Boston biotechnology community, *Organization Science*, 15(1): 5–21.

Pande, A. (2009), "It may be her eggs but it's my blood." Surrogates and everyday forms of kinship in India, *Qualitative Sociology*, 32: 379–397.

Pande, A. (2010), Commercial surrogacy in India: Manufacturing a perfect mother-worker, *Signs*, 35(4): 969–992.

Parsons, T. (1951), *The social system*, London and New York: Routledge.

Parsons, T. (1956), Suggestions for a sociological approach to the theory of organizations-I, *Administrative Science Quarterly*, 1: 63–85.

Partnoy, F. (1999), The Siskel and Ebert of financial markets?: Two thumbs down for the credit rating agencies, *Washington University Law Quarterly*, 77(3): 619–714.

Paruchuri, S. (2010), Intraorganizational networks, interorganizational networks, and the impact of central inventors. A longitudinal study of pharmaceutical firms, *Organization Science*, 21(1): 63–80.

Pascal, B. (1966), *Pensées*, London: Penguin.

Peet, R. (2011), Inequality, crisis and austerity in finance capitalism, *Cambridge Journal of Regions, Economy and Society*, 4(3): 383–399.

Pentland, B.T. (2000), Will auditors take over the world? Programs, techniques, and verification of everything, *Accounting, Organization & Society*, 25: 307–312.

Perlow, L. (1998), Boundary control: The social ordering of work and family time in high-tech corporation, *Administrative Science Quarterly*, 43(2): 328–357.

Perlow, L.A. (1999), The time famine: Toward a sociology of work time, *Administrative Science Quarterly*, 44: 57–81.

Péteri, G. (1989), Engineer utopia: On the position of technostructure in Hungary's war communism, 1919, *International Studies in Management & Organization*, 19(3): 82–102.

Pettigrew, A.M. (1973), *The politics of organizational decision-making*, London: Tavistock.

Pfeffer, J. and Salancik, G.R. (1978), *The external control of organizations: A resource dependence perspective*, New York: Harper and Row.

Pfeffer, N. (1999), *The stork and the syringe*, Cambridge: Polity.

Pickering, A. (1993), The mangle of practice: Agency and the emergence in the sociology of science, *American Journal of Sociology*, 99(3): 559–589.

Pickersgill, M. (2013), How personality became treatable: The mutual constitution of clinical knowledge and mental health law, *Social Studies of Science*, 43(1): 30–53.

Pitts-Taylor, V. (2007), *Surgery junkies: Wellness and pathology in cosmetic culture*, New Brunswick: Rutgers University Press.

Pitts-Taylor, V. (2010), The plastic brain: Neoliberalism and the neuronal self, *Health*, 14(6): 635–652.

Plato (1995), *Phaedrus*, Indianapolis and Cambridge: Hackett Publishing.

Polillo, S. and Guillén, M.F. (2005), Globalization pressures and the state: The worldwide spread of central bank independence, *American Journal of Sociology*, 110(6): 1764–1802.

Pottage, A. (2011), Law machines: Scale models, forensic materiality, and the making of modern patent law, *Social Studies of Science*, 41(5): 621–643.

Powell, W.W., Koput, K.W., White, D.R., and Owen-Smith, J. (2005), Network dynamics and field evolution: The growth of interorganizational collaboration in the life sciences, *American Journal of Sociology*, 110(4): 1132–1205.

Power, M. (1997), *The audit society: Rituals of verification*, Oxford and New York: Oxford University Press.

Power, M.K. (2003), Auditing and the production of legitimacy, *Accounting, Organization and Society*, 28: 379–394.

Preda, A. (2006), Socio-technical agency in financial markets: The case of the stock ticker, *Social Studies of Science*, 36: 753–782.

Purdy, J.M. and Grey, B. (2009), Conflicting logics, mechanisms of diffusion, and multilevel dynamics in emerging institutional fields, *Academy of Management Journal*, 52(2): 355–380.

Rabinow, P. (2003), *Anthropos today: Reflections on modern equipment*, Princeton and Oxford: Princeton University Press.

Rader, K.A. (2004), *Making mice: Standardizing animals for American biomedical research*, Princeton: Princeton University Press.

Rapp, R. (2011), Reproductive entanglements: Body, state, and culture in the dys/regulation of child-bearing, *Social Research*, 78(3).

Reay, T. and Hinings, C.R. (2009), Managing the rivalry of competing institutional logics, *Organization Studies*, 30(6): 629–652.

Rheinberger, H.-J. (1997), *Toward a history of epistemic things: Synthesizing proteins in the test tube*, Stanford: Stanford University Press.

Rheinberger, H.-J. (2000), Beyond nature and culture: Modes of reasoning in the age of molecular biology and medicine, in Lock, M., Youg, A., and Cambrosio, A., eds., (2000), *Living and working with new medical technologies: Intersections of inquiry*, Cambridge: Cambridge University Press, pp. 19–30.

Rheinberger, H.-J. (2010), *The epistemology of the concrete: Twentieth-century histories of life*, Durham and London: Duke University Press.

Robertson, J.A. (2010), Commerce and regulation in the assisted reproduction industry, in Goodwin, Michele Bratcher, ed., (2010), *Baby markets: Money and the new politics of creating families*, Cambridge: Cambridge University Press, pp. 191–207.

Rock, E.A. (2013), Adapting to the new shareholder-centric reality, *University of Pennsylvania Law Review*, 161(7): 1907–1988.

Roe, M. (2003), *Political determinants of corporate governance: Political context, corporate impact*, New York and Oxford: Oxford University Press.

Rorty, R. (1989), *Contingency, Irony, and Solidarity*, Cambridge: Cambridge University Press.

Rose, N.S. (2007), *The politics of life itself: Biomedicine, power and subjectivity in the twenty-first century*, Princeton and Oxford: Princeton University Press.

Ross, S.A. (1973), The economic theory of agency: The principal's problem, *American Economic Review*, 63: 134–139.

Roth, W.-M. (2005), Making classifications (at) work: Ordering practices in science, *Social Studies of Science*, 35(4): 581–621.

Roy, W.G. (1997), *Socializing capital: The rise of the large industrial corporation in America*, Princeton: Princeton University Press.

Rubin, B.P. (2008), Therapeutic promise in the discourse of human embryonic stem cell research, *Science as Culture*, 17(1): 13–27.

Salter, B. and Salter, C. (2007), Bioethics and the global moral economy: The cultural politics of human embryonic stem cell science, *Science, Technology and Human Values*, 32(5): 554–581.

Sayes, E. (2014), Actor-network theory and methodology: Just what does it mean to say that nonhumans have agency?, *Social Studies of Science*, 44(1): 134–149.

Schmidt, R., Sage, D., Eguchi, T., and Dainty, A. (2012), Moving architecture and flattening politics: Examining adaptability through a narrative of design, *Architectural Research Quarterly*, 16(1): 75–84.

Schor, J.B. (1993), *The overworked American*, New York: Basic Books.

Schrödinger, E. (1946), *What is life?: Physical aspects of the living cell*, Cambridge: Cambridge University Press.

Schumpeter, J.A. (1942), *Capitalism, socialism, and democracy*, New York: Harper & Row.

Scott, W.R. (2008), Lords of the dance: Professionals as institutional agents, *Organization Studies*, 29(2): 219–238.

Searle, J.R. (1995), *The construction of social reality*, London: Penguin.

Selin, C. (2007), Expectations and the emergence of nanotechnology, *Science, Technology & Human Values*, 32(2): 196–220.

Sell, S.K. (2003), *Private power, public law: The globalization of intellectual property rights*, New York: Cambridge University Press.

Selznick, P. (1949), *TVA and the grassroots*, Berkeley: University of California Press.

Selznick, P. (1996), Institutionalism "old" and "new," *Administrative Science Quarterly*, Vol. 40, June, pp. 270–277.

Serres, M. (1982), *The parasite*, Baltimore: John Hopkins University Press.

Sewell Jr, W.H. (1992), A theory of structure: Duality, agency, and transformation, *American Journal of Sociology*, 98(1), 1–29.

Sharp, L.A. (2003), *Strange harvest: Organ transplants, denatured bodies, and the transformed self*, Berkeley: University of California Press.

Sharp, L.A. (2007), *Bodies, commodities, and biotechnologies: Death, mourning, and scientific desire in the realm of human organ transfer*, New York: Columbia University Press.

Sharp. L.A. (2011), The invisible woman: The bioaesthetics of engineered bodies, *Body & Society*, 17(1): 1–30.

Shaw, J. (2012), The *Birth of the clinic* and the advent of reproduction: Pregnancy, pathology and the medical gaze in modernity, *Body & Society*, 18(2): 110–138.

Shostak, S. and Conrad, P. (2008), Sequencing and its consequences: Path dependence and the relationships between genetics and medicalization, *American Journal of Sociology*, 114: S287–S316.

Simmel, G. (1984), *On women, sexuality and love*, trans. by Guy Oakes, New Haven and London: Yale University Press.

Simondon, G. ([1958] 1980), *On the mode of existence of technical objects*, trans. by Ninian Mallahphy, London: University of Western Ontario.

Simonds, W. (1996), *Abortion at work: Ideology and practice in a feminist clinic*, New Brunswick: Rutgers University Press.

Singer, D.A. (2007), *Regulating capital: Setting standards for the international financial system*, Ithaca and London: Cornell University Press.

Siraisi, N.G. (2012), Medicine, 1450–1620, and the history of science, *Isis*, 103: 491–514.

Smerdon, U.R. (2008), Crossing bodies, crossing borders: International surrogacy between the United States and India, *Cumberland Law Review*, 39: 15–85.

Snowdon, C. (1994), What makes a mother? Interviews with women involved in egg donation and surrogacy, *Birth*, 21(2): 77–84.

Solow, R.M. (1957), Technical change and the aggregate production function, *The Review of Economics and Statistics*, 39(3): 312–320.

Spar, D. (2006), *The baby business: How money, science, and politics drive the commerce of conception*, Boston: Harvard Business School Press.

Spar, D.L. (2010), Free markets, free choice? A market approach to reproductive rights, in Goodwin, Michele Bratcher, ed., (2010), *Baby markets: Money and the new politics of creating families*, Cambridge: Cambridge University Press, pp. 177–190.

Spradley, J.P. (1979), *The ethnographic interview*, New York: Holt, Rineharrt and Winston.

Stake, R.E. (1996), *The art of case study research*, Thousand Oaks, London and New Delhi: Sage.

Star, S.L. (1999), The ethnography of infrastructure, *American Behavioral Scientist*, 43(3): 377–391.

Stark, David, (2009), *The sense of dissonance: Accounts of worth in economic life*, Princeton: Princeton University Press.

Stiegler, B. (2011), *Technics and time, 3: Cinematic time and the question of malaise*, Stanford: Stanford University Press.

Stigler, G.J. (1971), The theory of economic regulation, *Bell Journal of Economics and Management Science*, 2(1): 3–21.

Stiglitz, J.E. (2010), *Freefall: America, free markets, and the sinking of the world economy*, New York and London: WW. Norton.

Stinchcombe, A.L. (1997), On the virtue of the old institutionalism, *Annual Review of Sociology*, 23: 1–18.

Stout, L.A. (2012), *The shareholder value myth: How putting shareholders first harms investors, corporations and the public*, San Francisco: Berrett-Koehler.

Stout, L.A. (2013), Toxic side effects of shareholder primacy, *University Pennsylvania Law Review*, 161(7): 2003–2023.

Stryker, R. (2003), Mind the gap: Law, institutional analysis and socioeconomics, *Socio-Economic Review*, 1(3): 335–367.

Styhre, A. (2015), *Life science innovation: Venture capital, corporate governance and commercialization*, Basingstoke and New York: Palgrave Macmillan.

Styhre, A. and Tienari, J. (2013), Self-reflexivity scrutinized: (Pro-)feminist men learning that gender matters, *Equality, Diversity and Inclusion*, 32(2): 195–210.

Styhre, A., Wikmalm, L., Ollila, S., and Roth, J. (2012), Sociomaterial practices in engineering work: The backtalk of materials and the tinkering of resources, *Journal of Engineering, Design and Technology*, 10(2): 151–167.

Suchman, L.A. (2007), *Human–machine reconfigurations: Plans and situated actions*, Cambridge: Cambridge University Press.

Suddaby, R. (2006), From the editors: What grounded theory is not, *Academy of Management Journal*, 49(4): 633–642.

Suddaby, R. and Viale, T. (2011), Professionals and field-level change: Institutional work and the professional project, *Current Sociology*, 59(4): 423–444.

Suddaby, R., Hardy, C., and Huy, Q. (2011), Where are the new theories of organization?, *Academy of Management Review*, 36(2): 236–246.

Sunder Rajan, K. (2006), *Biocapital: The constitution of postgenomic life*, Durham: Duke University Press.

Sunder Rajan, K. (2012), Introduction: The capitalization of life and the liveliness of capital, in Sunder Rajan, K., ed., (2012), *Lively capital*, Durham and London: Duke University Press, pp. 1–41.

Sutton, J., Dobbin, F., Meyer, J.W., and Scott, W.R. (1994), The legalization of the workplace, *American Journal of Sociology*, 99: 944–971.

Tabb, W.J. (2012), *The restructuring of capitalism*, New York: Columbia University Press.

Taylor, J.S. (2005), Surfacing the body's interior, *Annual Review of Anthropology*, 34: 741–756.

Teman, E. (2010), *Birthing a mother: The surrogate body and the pregnant self*, Berkeley, Los Angeles and London: University of California Press.

Thacker, E. (2010), *After life*, Chicago and London: The University of Chicago Press.

Thomas, T.C. and Acuña-Narvaez, R. (2006), The convergence of biotechnology and nanotechnology: Why here, why now?, *Journal of Commercial Biotechnology*, 12(2): 105–110.

Thompson, J.D. (1967), *Organizations in Action*, New York: McGraw-Hill.

Thornton, P.H. (2002), The rise of the corporation in a craft industry: Conflict and conformity in institutional logics, *Academy of Management Journal*, 45: 81–101.

Thornton, P.H. and Ocasio, W. (2008), Institutional logics, in Greenwood, R., Oliver, C., Sahlin, K. and Suddaby, R., eds., (2008), *The Sage handbook of organizational institutionalism*, London, Thousand Oaks and New Delhi: Sage, pp. 99–129.

Titmuss, R.M. (1970), *The gift relationship: From human blood to social policy*, London: George Allen and Unwin.

Tober, D.M. (2001), Semen as gift, semen as good: Reproductive workers and the market in altruism, *Body & Society*, 7(2–3): 137–160.

Tomaskovic-Devey, D. and Lin, K.-H. (2011), Income dynamics, economic rents, and the financialization of the U.S. economy, *American Sociological Review*, 76(4): 538–559.

Townley, B. (2008), *Reason's neglect: Rationality and organizing*, Oxford and New York: Oxford University Press.

Trigilia, C. (2002), *Economic sociology: State, market, and society in modern capitalism*, Malden: Blackwell.

Tversky, A. and Kahneman, D. (1981), The framing of decisions and the psychology of choice, *Science*, 211(4481): 453–458.

Twine, F.W. (2011), *Outsourcing the womb: Race, class and gestational surrogacy in a global market*, London and New York: Routledge.

Van Arnum, B.M. and Naples, M.I. (2013), Financialization and Income Inequality in the United States, 1967–2010, *American Journal of Economics and Sociology*, 72(5): 1158–1182.

Van der Zwan, N. (2014), Making sense of financialization, *Socio-Economic Review*, 12(1): 99–129.

Van Maanen, J. (1979), The fact of fiction in organizational ethnography, *Administrative Science Quarterly*, 24: 539–550.

Van Maanen, J. (2011), Ethnography as work: Some rules of engagement, *Journal of Management Studies*, 48: 218–234.

Velthuis, O. (2007), *Talking prices: Symbolic meanings of prices on the market for contemporary art*, Princeton and London: Princeton University Press.

Velthuis, O. (2011), Damien's dangerous idea: Valuing contemporary art, in Beckert, Jens and Aspers, Patrik, eds., (2011), *The worth of goods: Valuation and pricing in the economy*, Princeton: Princeton University Press, pp. 178–200.

Vogel, S.K., (1996), *Freer markets, more rules: Regulatory reforms in advanced industrial countries*, Ithaca and London: Cornell University Press.

Waldby, C. (2002), Stem cells, tissue cultures, and the production of biovalue, *Health*, 6(3): 305–322.

Waldby, C. and Mitchell, R. (2006), *Tissue economies: Blood, organs, and cell lines in late capitalism*, Durham and London: Duke University Press.

Wallerstein, I.M. (2011), *The modern world system 4: 1879–1914*, Berkeley, Los Angeles and London: University of California Press.

Watkins, E.S. (2001), *On the pill: A social history of oral contraceptives, 1950–1970*, Baltimore and London: Johns Hopkins University Press.

Watson, T.J. (2011), Ethnography, reality, and truth: The vital need for studies of how things work organizations and management, *Journal of Management Studies*, 48: 202–217.

Watts, J.H. (2009), "Allowed into a man's world" meanings of work-life balance: Perspectives on women civil engineers as "minority" workers in construction, *Gender, Work and Organization*, 16(1): 37–57.

Weber, M. (1948), Science as a vocation, in *From Max Weber: Essays in sociology*, Ed. by H.H. Gerth and C. Wright Mills, London: Routledge and Kegan Paul, pp. 129–156.

Weber, M. (1949), *The methodology of the social sciences*, New York: Free Press.

White, H. (1987), *The content of form: Narrative discourse and historical representation*, Baltimore and London: Johns Hopkins University Press.

Whittington, K.B., Owen-Smith, J., and Powell, W.W. (2009), Networks, propinquity and innovation in knowledge-intensive industries, *Administrative Science Quarterly*, 54: 90–112.

Wynne, B. (2005), Reflexing complexity: Post-genomic knowledge and reductionist returns in public science, *Theory, Culture & Society*, 22(5): 67–94.

Yakubovich, V., Granovetter, M., and McGuire, P. (2005), Electric charges: The social construction of rate systems, *Theory and Society*, 34: 579–612.

Yates, J. (1989), *Control through communication*, Baltimore and London: The Johns Hopkins University Press.

Yue, L.Q., Luo, J. and Ingram, P. (2013), The failure of private regulation: Elite control and market crises in the Manhattan banking industry, *Administrative Science Quarterly*, 58(1): 37–68.

Zelizer, V. (1985), *Pricing the priceless child: The changing social value of children*, New York: Basic Books.

Zelizer, V. (2005), *The purchase of intimacy*, Princeton: Princeton University Press.

Zelizer, V. (2011), *Economic lives: How culture shapes the economy*, Princeton and Oxford: Princeton University Press.

Zorn, D.M. (2004), Here a chief, there a chief: The rise of the CFO in the American firm, *American Sociological Review*, 69: 345–364.

Zorn, D., Dobbin, F., Dierkes, J., and Kwok, M. (2005), Managing investors: How financial markets reshaped the American firm, in Knorr Cetina, Karin and Preda, Alex, eds., (2005), *The sociology of financial markets*, Oxford and New York: Oxford University Press. pp. 269–289.

Zweiger, G. (2001), *Transducing the genome: Information, anarchy and revolution in the biomedical sciences*, New York: McGraw-Hill.

Index